Soft Workouts

Low-Impact Exercise

Fitness, Health & Nutrition was created by Rebus, Inc. and published by Time-Life Books.

REBUS, INC.

Publisher: RODNEY FRIEDMAN
Editorial Director: CHARLES L. MEE JR.

Editor: THOMAS DICKEY
Executive Editor: SUSAN BRONSON
Senior Editor: MARY CROWLEY
Associate Editors: WILLIAM DUNNETT, CARL LOWE
Copy Editor: LINDA EPSTEIN
Contributing Editor: JACQUELINE DAMIAN

Art Director: JUDITH HENRY
Designer: FRANCINE KASS
Photographer: STEVEN MAYS
Photo Stylist: NOLA LOPEZ
Photo Assistant: TIMOTHY JEFFS

Test Kitchen Director: GRACE YOUNG
Recipe Editor: BONNIE J. SLOTNICK
Contributing Editor: MARYA DALRYMPLE
Chief of Research: CARNEY W. MIMMS III
Assistant Editor: PENELOPE CLARK

Time-Life Books Inc. is a wholly owned subsidiary of

TIME INCORPORATED

Founder: HENRY R. LUCE 1898-1967

Editor-in-Chief: JASON MCMANUS
Chairman and Chief Executive Officer: J. RICHARD MUNRO
President and Chief Operating Officer: N.J. NICHOLAS JR.
Corporate Editor: RAY CAVE
Executive Vice President, Books: KELSO F. SUTTON
Vice President, Books: GEORGE ARTANDI

TIME-LIFE BOOKS INC.

Editor: GEORGE CONSTABLE

Executive Editor: ELLEN PHILLIPS
Director of Design: LOUIS KLEIN
Director of Editorial Resources: PHYLLIS K. WISE
Editorial Board: RUSSELL B. ADAMS JR., DALE M. BROWN,
ROBERTA CONLAN, THOMAS H. FLAHERTY, LEE HASSIG,
DONIA ANN STEELE, ROSALIND STUBENBERG,
KIT VAN TULLEKEN, HENRY WOODHEAD
Director of Photography and Research: JOHN CONRAD
WEISER

President: CHRISTOPHER T. LINEN
Chief Operating Officer: JOHN M. FAHEY JR.
Senior Vice President: JAMES L. MERCER
Vice Presidents: STEPHEN L. BAIR, RALPH J. CUOMO,
NEAL GOFF, STEPHEN L. GOLDSTEIN, JUANITA T. JAMES,
HALLETT JOHNSON III, CAROL KAPLAN, SUSAN J.
MARUYAMA, ROBERT H. SMITH, PAUL R. STEWART,
JOSEPH J. WARD
Director of Production Services: ROBERT J. PASSANTINO

Editorial Operations
Copy Chief: DIANE ULLIUS
Production: CELIA BEATTIE
Library: LOUISE D FORSTALL

Soft Workouts

Low-Impact Exercise

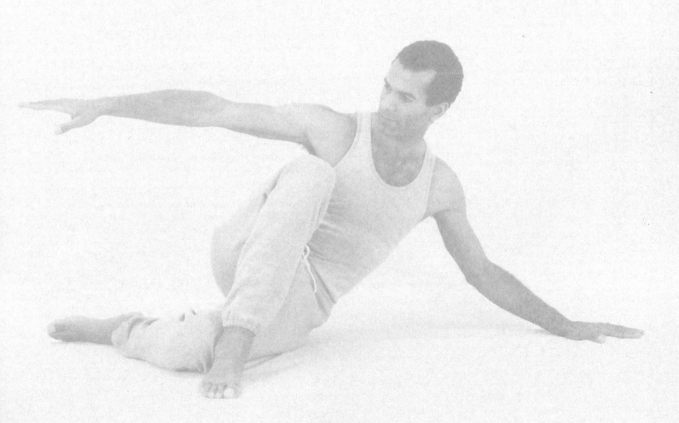

Time-Life Books, Alexandria, Virginia

CONSULTANTS FOR THIS BOOK

Robert M. Otto, Ph.D., is Director of the Human Performance Laboratory at Adelphi University, Garden City, N.Y. He is a member of the American College of Sports Medicine's Preventive and Rehabilitative Exercise Program Committee and of the Fitness Instructor Subcommittee, which is responsible for the development of Dance Exercise Certification.

Ann Grandjean, Ed.D., is Associate Director of the Swanson Center for Nutrition, Omaha, Neb.; chief nutrition consultant to the U.S. Olympic Committee; and an instructor in the Sports Medicine Program, Orthopedic Surgery Department, University of Nebraska Medical Center.

Myron Winick, M.D., is the R.R. Williams Professor of Nutrition, Professor of Pediatrics, Director of the Institute of Human Nutrition, and Director of the Center for Nutrition, Genetics and Human Development at Columbia University College of Physicians and Surgeons. He has served on the Food and Nutrition Board of the National Academy of Sciences and is the author of many books, including *Your Personalized Health Profile*.

The following consultants helped design the exercise sequences in this book:

Risa Friedman has a master's degree in dance education and is certified in health fitness by the American College of Sports Medicine, the International Dance Exercise Association and the Laban-Bartenieff Institute of Movement Studies. She has taught anatomy/kinesiology, movement analysis, therapeutic exercise, exercise physiology, and fitness and dance at New York University and the State University of New York, among other institutions. She is an exercise physiologist in private practice in San Diego, California, and is Program Director of the Fitness Specialist Certification Program at Marymount Manhattan College in New York City.

Jane Katz, Ed.D., is a Professor of Health and Physical Education, Bronx Community College of the City University of New York. An All-American Masters swimmer and synchronized swimming champion, Katz holds several World and National Masters swimming records. She is also a recipient of the National Fitness Leaders Award, given by the U.S. Jaycees and the President's Council on Physical Fitness.

Judy L. Marriott is a Certified Movement Analyst with the Laban-Bartenieff Institute of Movement Studies and an exercise trainer. She is also a professional dancer and has performed with several companies nationally and internationally.

Jean Ann Scharpf, M.A., is an exercise physiologist; Professor of Physical Education at Suffolk County Community College, Sheldon, N.Y.; and is certified as an exercise test technologist by the American College of Sports Medicine. As president of Shaping Routines, Inc., a fitness consulting firm, Scharpf is an aerobic and fitness instructor for educational, corporate and training workshops.

For information about any Time-Life book please write:
Reader Information
Time-Life Customer Service
P.O. Box C-32068
Richmond, Virginia 23261-2068

First printing.
Published simultaneously in Canada.
School and library distribution by Silver Burdett Company, Morristown, New Jersey.

TIME-LIFE is a trademark of Time Incorporated U.S.A.

Library of Congress Cataloging-in-Publication Data
Soft workouts.
(Fitness, health & nutrition)
Includes index.
1. Exercise. 2. Physical education and training. 3 Physical fitness. 4. Nutrition.
I. Time-Life Books. II. Series: Fitness, health and nutrition.
GV461.S62   1988   613.7′1   87-33604
ISBN 0-8094-6195-1
ISBN 0-8094-6196-X (lib. bdg.)

This book is not intended as a substitute for the advice of a physician. Readers who have or suspect they may have specific medical problems, especially those involving muscles and joints, should consult a physician before beginning any program of strenuous physical exercise.

CONTENTS

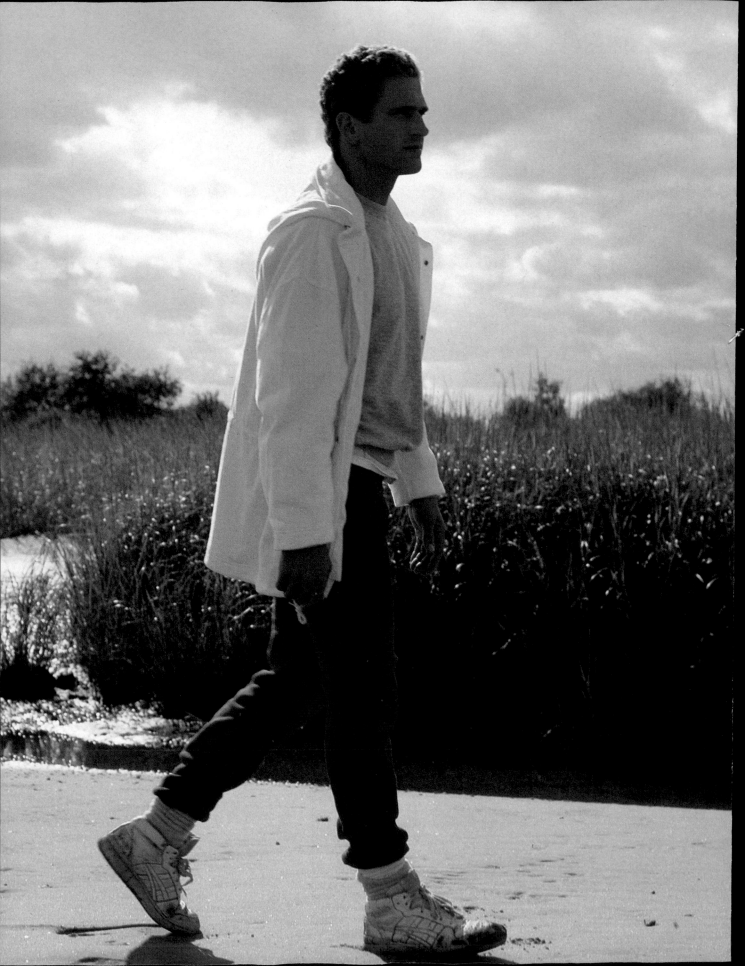

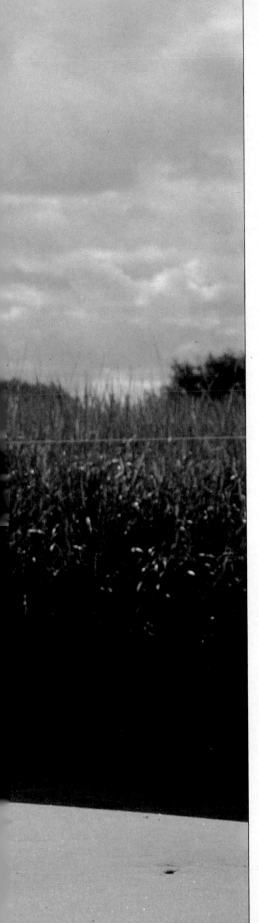

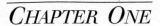

CHAPTER ONE

Soft Fitness

Reducing the impact of exercise to prevent injury, maintain health benefits and increase enjoyment

As exercise programs proliferate and research on them gains in sophistication, the standards of what makes exercise beneficial are changing. The notion that a workout should be painful or exhausting — that it should "burn" — has lost its validity, and a growing number of doctors and physiologists affirm that more moderate forms of exercise, which fall under the umbrella term "soft workouts," can improve fitness. One reason for this move toward gentler exercise is the rising incidence of injuries associated with some popular activities, particularly aerobic dance and running. Making soft workouts a part of your fitness program can be beneficial, since fewer stressful movements reduce the risk of injuries. But equally important, such exercises are accessible to people who are intimidated by — or who have tried and given up on — highly strenuous regimens. A crucial aspect of any exercise is that it be performed regularly. In providing a series of safe, effective and enjoyable routines, this book will help you toward that goal.

What is a soft workout?

Any exercise that minimizes the stress placed on the body's musculoskeletal system can be considered a soft workout. Also known as low-impact or low-percussive exercise, this type of workout provides an alternative to such exercise as high-impact aerobic dance and running — two activities that are considered high in the stress they place on the body, and yet are also among among the most popular forms of exercise, with some 40 million Americans participating in one or the other. In both running and traditional aerobic dance, you are airborne briefly, and the force of landing and taking off can jar your muscles, joints and ligaments, resulting in soreness or injury. Soft workouts dissipate such force by utilizing movements that enable you to keep one foot on the ground, and by offering such low-impact environments or surfaces as an exercise mat or a swimming pool.

What types of injuries do soft workouts help you avoid?

The injuries that committed exercisers tend to sustain are not usually of the obvious, acute kind, such as a sprained wrist or a fractured ankle. Rather, people who exercise regularly are more prone to stress, or overuse, injuries, which occur over time as a result of repeated strains on joints, bones and muscles. Typically, a stress injury occurs when the body is subjected to shock or impact while running or jumping, and the body's machinery does not absorb the force effectively. This can occur for a variety of reasons, including poor technique, inadequate equipment and biomechanical abnormalities — such as being flat-footed — that cause forces of exercise to be unevenly distributed through the musculoskeletal system. Though they are often less traumatic than acute injuries, stress injuries can take the form of a wide range of debilitating conditions, from the inflammation of muscles and tendons to muscle tears or hairline fractures in bones.

The rate of stress injuries varies for different activities. As many as 20 percent of joggers have to stop running for at least a week during each year because of running-related injuries. One in 10 runners suffers an injury each year — usually involving the knees, legs, hips and feet — that requires medical attention. A poll of aerobic dance teachers found that 75 percent of them, as well as 43 percent of their students, had suffered injuries as a result of their workouts.

For other activities whose movements produce less impact, injury rates are comparatively lower. Even swimmers can sustain stress injuries to the shoulder, however, and weight lifters, who neither jump nor run, are nonetheless prone to stress injuries. In order to lessen the risk of these injuries, anyone who exercises should take such preventive steps as properly warming up and cooling down, as well as increasing the intensity and frequency of workouts gradually. In addition, making soft workouts a part of your fitness program can be beneficial, since they minimize or eliminate the movements that

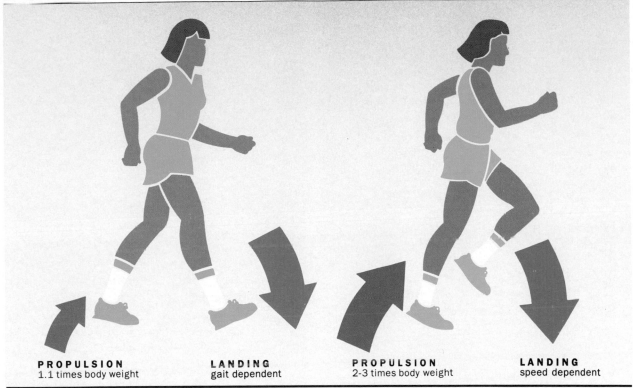

| PROPULSION
1.1 times body weight | LANDING
gait dependent | PROPULSION
2-3 times body weight | LANDING
speed dependent |

WALKING   **RUNNING**

create the greatest stress. Furthermore, low-impact routines also tend to raise your heart rate more gradually than high-impact exercises do; as a result, you are less likely to feel out of breath or prematurely fatigued if you are embarking on an exercise program.

Is "soft workouts" simply another term for low-impact aerobic dance?

By no means. Certainly low-impact aerobic dance is a popular and effective option for a soft workout. Some 70 percent of aerobic dance teachers who are members of the International Dance-Exercise Association have reported that they offer low-impact aerobic classes to help participants avoid injuries. In these classes, dancers typically have at least one foot on the floor at all times and move their arms constantly — swinging, doing biceps curls, overhead arm presses and so on. These arm movements help elevate the heart rate and promote aerobic activity that conditions the cardiovascular system. The aerobic dance routine in Chapter Two meets both of these criteria.

Many other types of exercise regimens besides low-impact aerobic movement are considered soft workouts. Fitness walking, which is

Both running and walking entail two phases: propulsion, or push-off, and landing. In running, the propulsive phase must exert enough force to propel the body off the ground; researchers now suspect that this phase can place as much stress on the foot as landing. Surprisingly, the landing phase of brisk walking can, depending on heel placement, be almost as stressful as that of running. However, the propulsive force is two to three times less in walking, since the body does not have to be launched into the air. This lesser force is what contributes significantly to the low-impact, low-injury quality of walking.

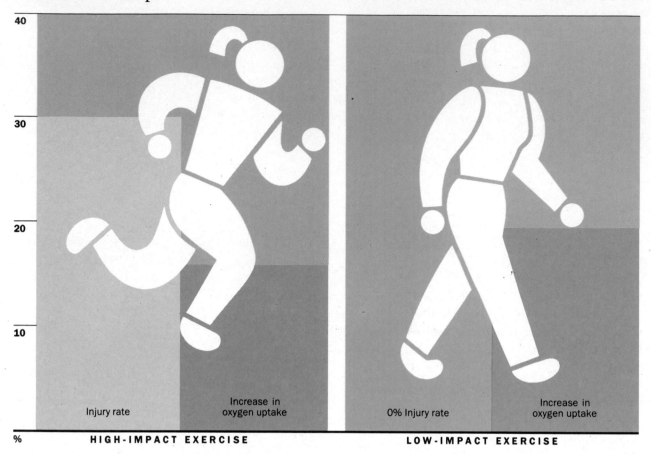

Injury rate	Increase in oxygen uptake
HIGH-IMPACT EXERCISE	

0% Injury rate	Increase in oxygen uptake
LOW-IMPACT EXERCISE	

A low-impact exercise like walking can provide the fitness benefits of high-impact routines like running without the risks. Two separate studies recorded fitness gains and injuries when groups of sedentary middle-aged women embarked on both low- and high-impact exercise programs. The women in the first study were on a jogging program, and nearly a third of them developed injuries *(left)*, mostly to the knee and leg. There were no injuries in the second study *(right)*, which involved brisk walking, water aerobics and other low-impact routines. The two groups achieved roughly the same improvement in VO$_2$max, a measure of how efficiently your body uses oxygen during intense exercise.

perhaps the fastest-growing form of exercise in the United States, is inherently low in impact and has a very low injury rate. Whereas both feet leave the ground during a running stride, you always have one foot on the ground when you walk. A section in Chapter Two shows you how to turn walking into a fitness exercise.

Other kinds of soft workouts — such as the routines in Chapter Three, which are performed in water — rely on the cushioning effect of the exercise medium to absorb the shock of movement. Another form of low-impact exercise consists of dancelike movement routines based on principles of kinesiology, the study of how the human body moves. Such routines, which are demonstrated in Chapter Four, can strengthen and tone muscles without undue jarring or strain.

Aren't soft workouts mainly for people who are injured or badly out of shape?
A number of soft workout routines are based on fitness programs developed for people who were recovering from injuries or who had some other condition — such as pregnancy or obesity — that kept them from participating in more taxing forms of exercise. As a result,

soft exercises are accessible to just about anyone, regardless of the participant's physical condition. At the same time, many highly fit people have also taken to softening their workouts as a means of injury prevention. Committed exercise enthusiasts who do not want to give up their high-impact programs are finding that they can integrate soft workouts into their usual routines and obtain the benefits of both. For example, researchers have found that running injuries increase in direct proportion to how often you run and also how far you run. A runner concerned with the possibility of being hurt and forced to lay off exercise might choose, therefore, to run three days a week rather than five and to walk, do water workouts or other low-impact aerobics on the other two days. Such a regimen minimizes the risk of injury while maintaining fitness and an active lifestyle. Even professional athletes are taking advantage of low-impact routines: A number of coaches report adding water based workouts to their teams' training regimens.

Highly trained women may find it especially valuable to alternate soft and hard workouts. Research has shown that strenuous exercise can produce undesirable hormonal changes. One report on female runners found that as many as half of all competitive runners have irregular menstrual cycles, and some actually stop menstruating. Some experts attribute this to lowered levels of the female hormone estrogen, which can lead to temporary infertility, and lowered calcium levels, which can sometimes cause a loss of bone tissue in the spine. These problems can be halted by cutting back the level of strenuous exercise.

But can soft workouts really exercise your heart intensely enough to be aerobic and improve your endurance?
Building cardiovascular endurance requires improving your oxygen consumption, or aerobic capacity, as this element of fitness is also known. Basically, oxygen consumption is the amount of oxygen that you can extract from the air and transport to working muscles for fuel. How much oxygen you consume is largely dependent on the efficiency of your cardiovascular system. For an exercise to affect oxygen consumption, it must employ large muscle groups like the legs and arms, and it must be continuous, to keep the demand for oxygen high.

Much of the research associated with the aerobic aspect of soft workouts has centered on walking — and virtually all of it shows that rapid walking can produce cardiovascular benefits in most people regardless of their level of fitness. In one study of 343 people spanning the ages of 30 to 69, fast walking enabled nearly all of the women and about two thirds of the men to reach their target heart rates. A person's target heart rate is a percentage of his or her maximum heart rate; it is one indicator that the heart is pumping hard enough during a workout — and that the workout itself is intense enough to be beneficial. As a person gets fitter, he or she must work harder to raise the heart rate because the heart is pumping more efficiently.

In order to see whether walking could continue to provide effective exercise as fitness levels increased, the same researchers also investigated whether a more highly fit population could obtain the same results. The outcome of this study — illustrated on page 15 — convinced them that walking can indeed build endurance and produce aerobic conditioning as long as the walkers keep to a pace commensurate with their fitness levels. And in a six-month study of middle-aged women who walked two miles a day, four days a week, the subjects attained aerobic and muscular improvements comparable to those of a traditional aerobic dance program.

A good deal of research is now being conducted on whether other types of low-impact workouts can also produce adequate cardiovascular benefits. The data accumulated thus far indicate that they can indeed. For example, one study compared the results of a group of 25 subjects who performed both high-impact and low-impact aerobic dance routines. Although the women's oxygen consumption rose 28 percent during the high-impact session, the heart-rate response during both sessions was nearly the same — the pulses recorded during the high-impact session averaged only eight percent higher than those in the low-impact session. The researchers concluded that while the high-impact routine provided a more intense workout, the low-impact program also provided an aerobic training stimulus — and that in fact it met the aerobic exercise guidelines set by the American College of Sports Medicine.

What other health benefits do soft workouts provide?

Like all forms of endurance exercise, soft workouts that exercise your heart and lungs can also help tone the skeletal muscles, especially those of the legs, hips, buttocks and abdomen. They have the ability to improve circulation and lung capacity, and can lower elevated blood pressure and reduce psychological stress. Also, several studies suggest that weight-bearing exercises like walking — that is, exercises that place mechanical stresses on the bone — can strengthen bone composition and slow down osteoporosis, a disease characterized by thinning and weakening of the bones.

What is perhaps the most impressive long-term benefit was revealed in a recent study of 35 male postal workers who had been walking an average of 25 miles a week for 15 to 28 years. The researchers found that this exercise had a beneficial effect on the subjects' cholesterol levels. The men, aged 36 to 58, had higher than average levels of HDL cholesterol, the good type of cholesterol-carrying lipoprotein that transports fats out of the bloodstream and thereby reduces the risk of heart disease. The link between long-term walking and increased HDL held up even after other factors — including age, leisure activities and alcohol consumption — were taken into consideration. Such a finding is significant because many sports physiologists have reported that, to increase HDL levels significantly, you need to run or perform some other intense aerobic exercise. This study appears to indicate that long-term, low-intensity exercise done regularly may provide the same benefit.

Can you achieve any fitness benefits from low-impact activities that do not qualify as complete workouts?

The health improvements that aerobic exercise can provide — lower blood pressure, greater cardiac efficiency, a sense of well-being, more energy, among others — can come only from sustained, regular exercise. But a long-term study conducted by the University of Minnesota showed that a moderate level of activity does have clear-cut advantages over a sedentary lifestyle. The subjects in the study were men at high risk for heart disease, and researchers found that men who engaged daily in such activities as gardening, dancing, home exercise and other so-called moderate exercise reduced the risk of a fatal heart attack by as much as one third over a seven-year period. Even for people who are not in a high-risk group, activities like bowling, golf and even doing domestic chores are a step toward better health.

Can you lose weight doing soft workouts?

Any exercise that burns calories will help you lose weight, and soft workouts are no exception. A number of studies support the view that soft routines are efficient calorie burners. For example, when 15 sedentary women between the ages of 35 and 64 undertook a 10-week program of low-impact aerobic dance, their body fat decreased by an average of 2.5 percent — without controlled dieting. In fact, in study after study, walking has been shown to be an excellent aid to weight control.

However, one researcher notes that you may have to work out longer to burn calories as effectively as those who are exercising more strenuously. In walking research, for example, physiologists have found that moderately brisk walking burns 1.15 calories per kilogram of body weight per mile, while running burns 1.7 calories. Roughly speaking, that means that you have to walk 1.5 miles to get the same caloric expenditure as running for one mile.

Can a mini-trampoline provide an effective workout?

Rebounding activity on a trampoline, which allows you to run and bounce with or without upper body movement, has been touted as a way to develop cardiovascular endurance; however, there is little evidence thus far to support the claims. Studies have shown minimal increases in aerobic fitness and no change in body composition in programs lasting from eight to 12 weeks. Other studies show no changes in HDL cholesterol levels.

Experts also acknowledge that a well-trained person will find it hard to reach his or her target heart rate by rebounding on a trampoline. The unconditioned individual can probably accomplish this goal, but with continued exercising the target heart rate will become more and more difficult to attain. One study did reveal some change in body weight — an average 12 percent decrease in overweight women. However, it is not uncommon for overweight individuals initially to lose some weight in most exercise programs, and there is no evidence that this weight would stay off if rebounding was the only exercise they performed persistently. Also, rebounding is not injury-free; there have been reports of painful, inflamed tendons associated with the bouncing.

What can movement routines add to a fitness program?
Movement routines are designed to improve body mechanics, the way you utilize and move your body. They accomplish this by focusing on basic maneuvers — like rolling over or rising from a sitting to a standing position — that make you conscious of all the muscles that contribute to performing these actions. This body awareness, in turn, helps you to move more effectively by building balance and coordination. The routines are extremely low in impact, and many of them incorporate stretching movements that will help to increase your flexibility, a further safeguard against injury.

Are water workouts as effective an exercise as swimming?
Swimming has long been touted as perhaps the single best form of exercise. It builds cardiovascular endurance superbly, develops muscle strength and boasts a very low injury rate. Water workouts are not intended to replace swimming, but they do offer the variety that lap swimming lacks, and they can be done by nonswimmers or by anyone whose swimming stroke is not efficient enough to enable him or her to swim laps.

Research also suggests that water workouts can be an effective and efficient aerobic conditioner. One study of college athletes working out in the water found that they were able to maintain their target heart rates and oxygen consumption during exercise sessions lasting up to 46 minutes. Another study compared target heart rates and other fitness measurements of 14 subjects who did walking and running tests on land and in the water. In the walking segments, their heart rates in the water were elevated about eight percent above the rates recorded on land. In the running segments, the heart rates were about equal in both tests — probably because of the difficulty of maintaining a brisk pace in the water. In addition, one researcher found that the greater resistance of water as compared to air creates an increased energy requirement of about 34 percent. As a result, you burn a third more calories performing an exercise in the water than you would performing the same exercise at the same pace on land.

Can you do water workouts and other soft routines while you are recovering from an injury?
Water has long been used for physical therapy and rehabilitation, and today more and more athletes and exercisers are taking advantage of

Hitting the Target Heart Rate

Heartbeats per minute

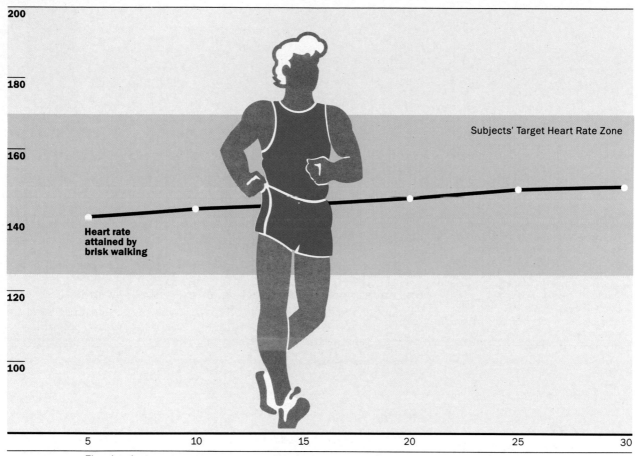

200

180

Subjects' Target Heart Rate Zone

160

140

Heart rate attained by brisk walking

120

100

5   10   15   20   25   30

Time in minutes

its healing qualities. Because of water's buoyancy, water exercises are nonweight-bearing, which means that they place no strain on the injured body part. Also, physiologists believe that water increases circulation, which speeds healing. Then, too, water has a soothing effect that can relieve pain. Other types of soft workouts can also help during recuperation from an injury. Often, an exerciser will choose a routine that is a softened version of his or her usual workout — an injured runner may get back in shape via a walking program, for example, or a high-impact aerobic dancer might shift to a low-impact movement routine.

How can you tell if you are working out at the proper intensity? The classic way is to take your pulse, which will tell you whether you are reaching your target heart rate. (For the formula on how to de-

Even highly fit exercisers can benefit from walking. In one study, male subjects who ranged in age from 22 to 39 were told to walk for half an hour at a pace that would enable each of them to reach his target heart rate — a rate that varies with age and that indicates a person is exercising intensely enough to obtain aerobic benefits. As shown above, all the subjects achieved this level of intensity after the first five minutes and maintained it for the rest of the walk.

Boosting the Workout

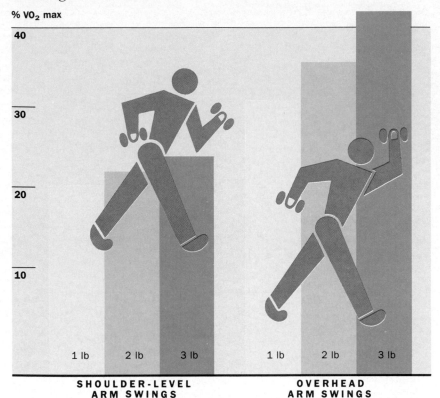

% VO$_2$ max

40

30

20

10

| 1 lb | 2 lb | 3 lb | | 1 lb | 2 lb | 3 lb |

SHOULDER-LEVEL ARM SWINGS   **OVERHEAD ARM SWINGS**

Swinging one's arms while carrying light hand weights can intensify a soft workout — and the more vigorous the arm swings, the better. One study examined the energy costs of walking workouts, as measured by VO$_2$max, when various-sized weights were added. All the workouts showed increases in VO$_2$max, but the change was most dramatic when the subjects walked while pumping their elbows up to ear level.

termine target heart rate, see page 21.) There are also two generally accepted rules of thumb. One is that if the workout makes you pant, you are working hard enough. The other rule is that you should be able to hold a conversation comfortably while exercising; if you are breathing so hard that speaking is difficult or impossible, you are probably working too hard.

Are there ways to boost the intensity of soft workouts?

Previously sedentary people who start a program of walking or another low-impact workout may quickly find themselves much improved in fitness. For them, and for people who are already well-trained yet want to soften their workouts for injury prevention, there are a number of ways to increase intensity to maintain continued effectiveness in improving fitness levels.

One method used in both walking and low-impact aerobic dance is to increase the work your arms are doing. One expert has calculated that keeping the arms in constant motion at shoulder level or above during exercise increases the heart rate enough to provide a moderate aerobic stimulus. In addition, many exercisers are relying on portable weights to increase the energy costs of their workouts.

Hand weights have been shown to modestly increase oxygen consumption, heart rate and the number of calories burned during exercise — usually by five to 10 percent. The most recent research suggests that the best approach to boosting your cardiovascular output is to combine controlled arm swinging and hand weights *(see illustration page 16)*. One study, for example, tested 20 men and women whose average age was 27, during normal walking, walking while vigorously swinging their arms, walking while carrying three-pound hand weights and walking plus arm swinging while equipped with the weights. The researchers found that only the combination of weights and vigorous arm swinging had a significant impact on oxygen consumption and heart rate; weights alone were insufficient to do this. (Most authorities urge caution when adding hand weights to your routine, especially if you are in less than optimal condition, have a history of heart disease or suffer from chronic musculoskeletal problems, particularly lower back pain.)

Backpacks, too, may produce a workload sufficient to increase conditioning in trained individuals, although the research results have been mixed. One study of 44 men aged 18 to 23 found that it was possible to improve the oxygen-uptake gains of a walking program by carrying 6 1/2-pound backpacks. However, another study found that in order to reach target heart rates, subjects had to carry an inordinate amount of baggage — the equivalent of some 40 percent of their body weight.

What kind of soft workout should you do?

One of the appealing features of soft workouts is that they provide you with a number of accessible, low-injury exercise options. Research has shown that boredom is a key factor in fitness drop-out rates, so variety in an exercise program is crucial. Many of the workouts here are interchangeable *(see chart page 23)* and can be tailored to your personal exercise preferences. For example, you might prefer indoor, low-impact aerobic dance in the winter, but switch to walking outside during the warmer months. This workout flexibility will encourage you to exercise more regularly, an essential element in attaining and maintaining fitness. To see how soft workouts can benefit you, turn the page.

F or quick, effective conditioning, try walking up and down stairs. Several work-site studies have found that people who began using stairs instead of elevators improved their fitness levels by 10 to 15 percent. Stair climbing is a good calorie burner, too: You may use 17.5 calories per minute if you climb two steps per second.

How to Design Your Own Program

You can use soft workouts in a variety of ways: as your primary form of exercise, as an exercise substitute during recovery from an injury or as a supplement to high-impact exercise. Additionally, you can alternate the different soft workouts themselves to provide your fitness program with variety. This quiz, and the remaining pages in this chapter, will help you to determine how much exercise is appropriate for your level of fitness, as well as which soft workouts are most suitable for your exercise needs.

Can you benefit from low-impact exercise?

1 Do you suffer occasional — or chronic — sports-related injuries?

Keeping injuries to a minimum is probably the most common reason for switching from a high-impact to a low-impact exercise program. Indeed, it was the excessive rates of injury in many high-impact exercises that led to the development of low-impact alternatives. For example, water workouts are actually an offspring of hydrotherapy — rehabilitative exercise programs in the water for injured or disabled persons. Because the risk of injury is greatly reduced in low-impact exercise, you are less likely to have to halt your workouts to allow for rest and recuperation. The more consistently you can exercise, the better able you will be to maintain your desired level of fitness. And even if you have to stop a high-impact exercise temporarily because of an injury, soft workouts can help maintain your conditioning so that you will have less difficulty getting up to speed when you are better.

2 Have you tried various forms of exercise, but repeatedly find yourself unable to stick to a program?

Exercise drop-out rates are a common problem. Physical drawbacks like injuries are only one of the difficulties; not having enough time or becoming bored after a few weeks or months can interfere with a workout program. Achieving fitness does demand a commitment of time and consistency of effort: To gain cardiovascular benefits from aerobic exercise, you must work out in your target heart range for at least 20 minutes three times a week, plus five minutes each of warm-ups and cool-downs. Similarly, strength training and exercising to improve your flexibility require workouts three or four times a week.

Soft workouts provide several different options to suit your personal preferences; you can alternate among them for variety. Walking, in particular, can easily be fit into any schedule and will allow you to achieve fitness benefits anytime and anywhere. That is why more and more people — including many who have not exercised in years — are joining the ranks of walkers.

3 Are you overweight?

Soft workouts can benefit anyone, but one of their primary advantages is that they are appropriate for overweight individuals, pregnant women or others who for health reasons should not perform heavy weight-bearing exercises. If you are overweight or have a musculoskeletal problem like weak knees or ankles, the pounding of high-impact exercise such as running and aerobic dance is even more damaging. Because soft workouts reduce or eliminate such impact, they can provide a safe exercise alternative for those for whom more stressful routines are inadvisable.

4 How far do you live from your workplace?

Walking is perhaps the ultimate low-impact exercise, in part because it can so easily be incorporated into the busiest schedule. And the fitness benefits of building exercise into your daily life might even protect against heart disease. A recent report issued by the Centers for Disease Control conclusively linked cardiac disease to a sedentary lifestyle; in fact, non-exercisers have almost double the risk of coronary disease as their more fit counterparts. Researchers at the centers suggest a regular schedule of moderate exercise like walking. Another study suggests that those who seek optimum cardiovascular fitness to help to increase their longevity should expend 2,000 calories weekly in physical activity, the equivalent of walking briskly about one hour a day, five times weekly.

To fit exercise into your existing schedule, try parking your car a mile or two from work, or getting off the bus or train several stops before your accustomed destination and walking the remainder of the way. A brisk walk at lunchtime is another convenient, easy way of working out.

5 Are your swimming abilities below average?

The natural buoyancy of water makes swimming one of the best low-impact exercise options, but you need not be a swimmer to achieve the benefits of exercising in this ideal low-impact environment. Water workouts simply take land exercises — such as running, sit-ups, stretches for flexibility — and adjust them for a swimming pool. Research has shown that these exercises have the same metabolic benefits in the water as on land. Indeed, the resistance of the water, which is almost 800 times heavier than air, can increase the effectiveness of some exercises — without increasing the stress on your musculoskeletal system.

6 Is a low-impact fitness program sufficient if you are already fit?

Low-impact exercise is not low-intensity exercise. Studies have shown that most people are able to achieve their target heart rates with fast walking. And low-impact aerobic dance is in some ways more difficult than high-impact as it requires greater coordination. (The movement routines on pages 102-123 will help increase your coordination and flexibility, and improve your ability to perform other types of exercise effectively.) However, if you are very fit, you might need to increase the effort of a soft workout by adding light hand weights while walking, dancing or working out in the water. Not only will this increase your heart rate, it will provide extra strengthening benefits.

Rating Your Fitness Level

To determine how fit you are at present and to monitor your progress during your exercise program, you can take the Rockport Fitness Walking Test at right. This test, which was developed for the Rockport Walking Institute by cardiologists and exercise scientists, is quite safe and can be taken by anyone. However, if you are over 35 years old, or if you have had any signs of heart disease, you should consult a physician before performing it. The test will give you a simple but accurate measurement of your cardiovascular endurance. The only equipment you need is a stopwatch to clock both your pulse and your one-mile walking time.

After taking the test, see how your results relate to the graph for your age and sex, at far right. You will fall into one of five fitness categories. If the results show that you are at a low or below average level of fitness, the workouts in this book help you improve your fitness level significantly.

As your fitness builds, or if you have already reached an average, above average or high level of fitness, you can increase the exertion of soft workouts by adding weights or following the other guidelines for intensifying exercise that are given in the following chapters. Take the test periodically — every month or two — to keep track of how your endurance is improving.

1-MILE WALK TEST

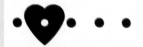

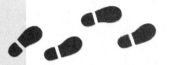

Step 1 Record your resting heart rate. Walk in place for 30 seconds, then use the tips of your second and third fingers to locate the radial artery in your wrist. First feel for the wristbone at the base of the thumb, then move your fingertips down your wrist until you find your pulse. Count your pulse for 15 seconds and multiply it by four to determine the rate per minute.

Step 2 Find a measured track or measure out a level mile. Then walk a mile as fast as you can. Record your time precisely at the end of the mile. (Walking speeds may vary in individuals, so you may want to repeat this test at a later date to make sure your first-mile time is typical for you.)

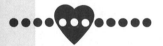

Step 3 Immediately record your heart rate at the end of the mile.

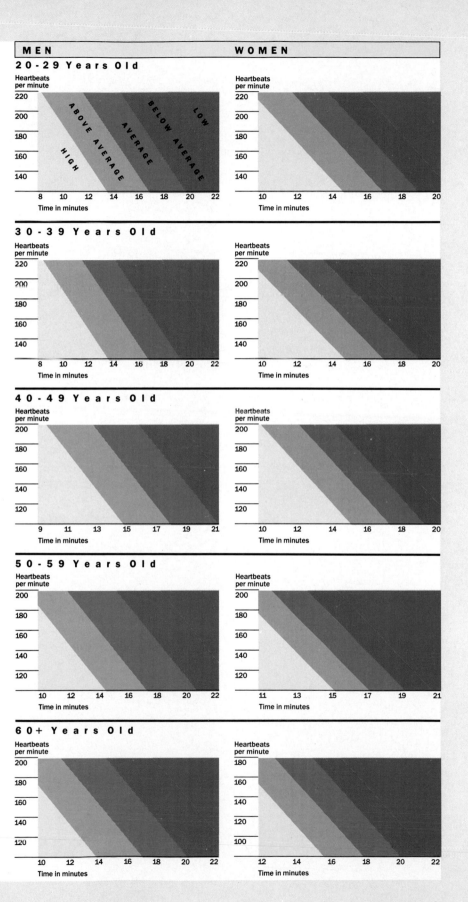

21

Choosing an Exercise

Soft workouts can encompass the four essential components of a fitness program, as the chart opposite indicates. This book provides endurance conditioning with low-impact aerobic exercises; muscle strengtheners that rely on light weights or are performed against water's resistance; nonballistic flexibility exercises; and movement routines that use the body's resistance to gravity to enhance coordination.

Some of the exercises on the following pages target more than one area of fitness. For example, walking with weights not only boosts your cardiovascular system, it also strengthens your arm muscles. How-ever, no single exercise provides benefits in all four categories. To get a comprehensive workout, you should perform exercises targeted at different fitness goals.

The soft workouts in the following three chapters provide several exercise options for each category of fitness. You may combine these components in various ways. For example, you might decide on a complete fitness program in the water. Or, you may prefer water workouts for strength and flexibility, a walking program for endurance and movement routines for coordination. Varying your set of exercises will keep your workouts interesting and challenging.

Targeting Your Workout

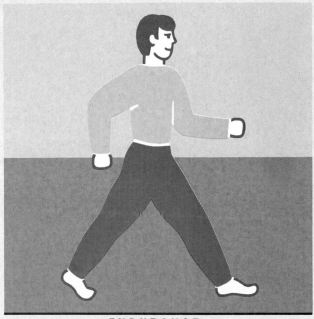

ENDURANCE

Aerobic exercise, which requires sustained activity that engages the large muscle groups of the body, stimulates the body's cardiovascular system and builds endurance.

low-impact dance *pages 36-53* **walking** *pages 64-69*
water workouts *pages 86-89*

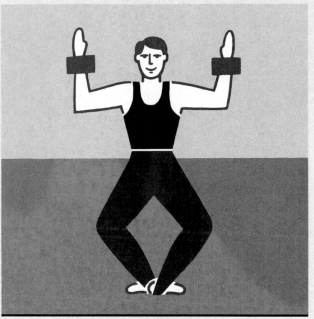

STRENGTH

Muscles grow stronger as greater demands are placed on them, either by increasing repetitions of a particular muscular action or by adding resistance—usually weights—to intensify the activity.

low-impact dance *pages 56-61* **walking** *pages 66-67*
water workouts *pages 76-81*

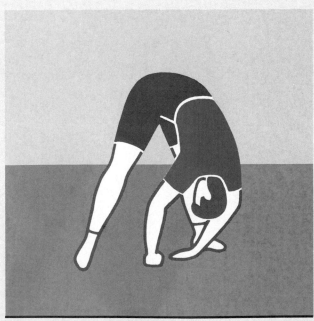

FLEXIBILITY

Flexibility is achieved through stretching exercises that develop the full range of motion in the muscles and joints. Stretching enhances your ability to perform exercises without injury and is an important component of warm-up routines.

water workouts *pages 82-85, 96-97* **movement** *pages 102-123*

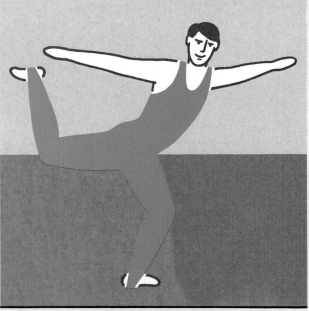

COORDINATION

Good coordination improves agility and is essential for the successful execution of any sport and most exercises. Moving your body in predetermined sequences that require concentration and body awareness helps develop this important aspect of fitness.

water workouts *pages 90-95* **movement** *pages 102-123*

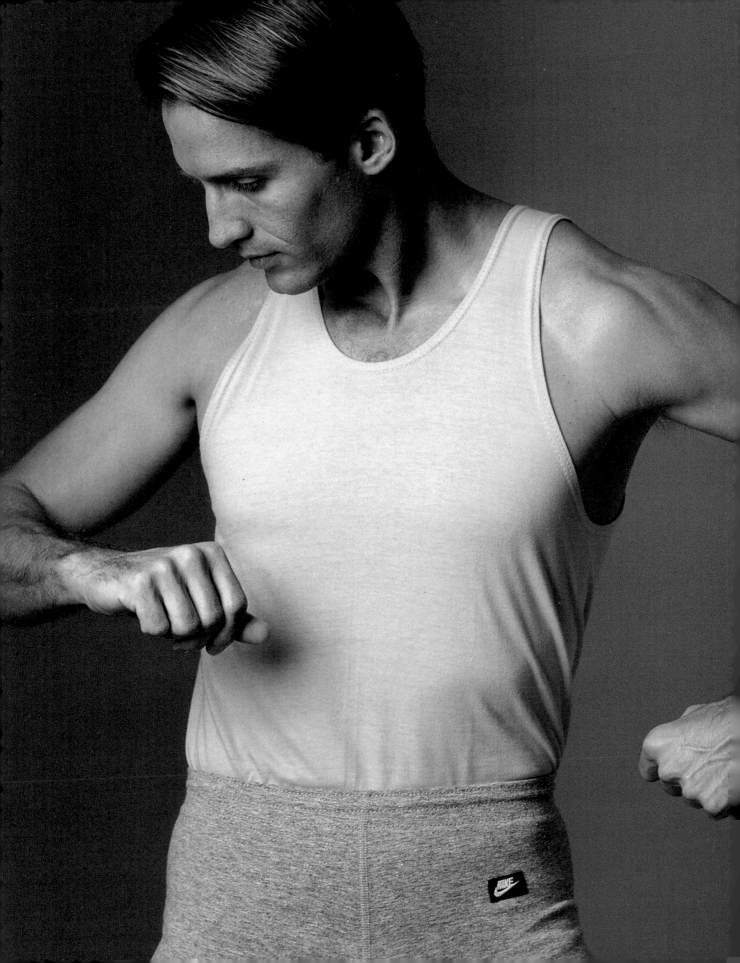

CHAPTER TWO

Aerobics

*The key: combining
arms and legs*

A erobic exercise, which uses repeated continuous, rhythmic movements of large muscle groups — primarily the arms and legs — to boost the cardiovascular system, forms the cornerstone of any fitness program. Low-impact aerobic exercise, which includes walking and aerobic dance, also encompasses such standard cardiovascular strengtheners as cycling, rowing and swimming.

When participants in low-impact dance and fitness walking programs exercise vigorously, they can reach and maintain their target heart rates for at least 20 minutes — the amount of time it takes to receive cardiovascular benefits from exercise, as determined by the American College of Sports Medicine. (To determine your target heart rate zone, subtract your age from 220. Multiply the remainder by .65 to determine the low end of the range and by .85 to calculate the high end. For cardiovascular conditioning, your pulse should fall between these two figures during aerobic exercise.) One study of middle-aged men found that those who walked 40 minutes a day, four days a week for 20 weeks showed cardiovascular improvements equal to participants in a 30-minute-a-day, three-times-a-week running program. A study of participants in aerobic dance classes indicated that they, too, achieved cardiovascular conditioning through regular workouts, with significant improvements after only six weeks.

The distinguishing feature of low-impact aerobic dance is that one foot always remains in contact with the floor. The jumping and bouncing inherent in high-impact aerobic dance — and at the root of most dance-related injuries — are replaced by walking, marching, side-stepping and lunging. An increase in upper-body work compensates for the reduced demands on the lower body. Because performing arm movements at or above the level of the heart helps boost your heart rate, vigorous but controlled arm work is essential.

Jumping in high-impact aerobics practically ensures that you will boost your heart rate. In contrast, the aerobic benefits of low-impact routines come from carefully choreographed combinations of arm and leg work. These routines must be performed with precision to achieve cardiovascular benefits, so low-impact routines require greater concentration and coordination than high-impact ones do.

To allow for the more deliberate coordination of low-impact dance, the music you use to pace yourself should be slightly slower — between 125 and 145 beats per minute — than it is for high-impact routines. If you are incorporating weights into your routine, choose music with a tempo of 120 to 140 beats per minute. Counting to the beat of the music will keep you working at the proper intensity as well as help you coordinate your movements.

Most injuries sustained in an aerobic dance program occur below the knee — shin splints, Achilles tendinitis and stress fractures. Reducing the impact lessens the stress on the lower body, but the increased lateral floor movements and arm use in low-impact routines can result in injuries to the back, shoulder, arms or knees. Taking a few precautions during your workout will minimize the risks. Maintain proper posture: abdominal muscles contracted, buttocks tucked under and knees slightly bent. When lunging, make sure that your bent knees never extend beyond your toes to avoid excess stress on ankle and knee ligaments; your knee should also always be pointed in the same direction as your lower leg. Be careful not to arch your back when working the upper body: Keeping your pelvis tilted forward and your knees relaxed will avoid this. Arm movements should be smooth and controlled; jerky arm movements can hyperextend and possibly injure the shoulder and elbow joints, forearms and wrists.

Like low-impact dance, walking is a grounded activity — one foot lands before the other pushes off. The foot rolls forward from heel landing to forefoot push-off, which spreads the propulsive and impact forces across a larger surface of the foot than running does (*see illustration page 10*). Day-to-day walking is usually performed at a two- to three-mile-per-hour pace. Depending on your level of condi-

Caring for Your Feet

Your feet, which contain 26 bones and more than 20 muscles, endure much of the stress of weight-bearing exercise — including walking and low-impact aerobic dance. Foot injuries associated with exercise range from simple blisters to painful heel spurs. Many such problems can be eliminated or reduced through proper foot care. The following suggestions will help you maintain the health of your feet and, in turn, exercise in greater comfort.

◆ Wear well-fitting shoes suited to your particular activity. Shoes that fit will feel comfortable as soon as you put them on; if you think they will need a break-in period, do not buy them. (For specific information on walking and aerobic shoes, turn the page.)

◆ Wash your feet daily with soap and warm water. Dry well, especially between the toes, an area prone to athlete's foot. Apply a nonlanolin moisturizing cream to dry skin on your heels or toes.

◆ Use foot powder. Apply an antifungal foot powder after cleaning your feet and also sprinkle it in your shoes to help absorb perspiration.

◆ Protect blister-prone areas on your feet with petroleum jelly before you exercise. If you do develop a large, painful blister, you can relieve the pressure by draining it: Cleanse it with an antiseptic solution and puncture around the edge with a sterile needle. Apply a topical antibiotic and cover. Keep your foot dry for a day or two to avoid infection.

◆ Do not treat other foot ailments yourself. Contact your doctor or podiatrist if you notice any persistent abrasion, rash or abnormality. Never try to cut away your own corns or bunions.

tioning, you need to walk between three and a half and four and a half miles per hour for optimum fitness. You must use your arms as you do in low-impact aerobic dance. Vigorous arm swinging will increase the effort demanded of walking, making it a fitness exercise.

As your aerobic fitness increases from either a walking or low-impact dance regimen, you will find that it becomes increasingly difficult for you to reach your target heart rate. This indicates that your heart muscle has adapted to the workload and become more efficient. Increasing movements that cross the floor and doing more arm work at shoulder level or higher will increase cardiovascular demands. You can further intensify your workouts by incorporating light hand-held or wrist weights. Adding weights, when combined with arm swinging, has been shown to increase oxygen consumption, heart rate and calories burned during exercise. Excluding warm-ups and cool-downs, you can use weights with any of the aerobic dance routines on the following pages. Exercises designed to strengthen particular muscles are shown on pages 56-61. Intensifying your walking program with weights is shown on pages 66-67. Retro, or backward, walking, demonstrated on pages 68-69, is a way to add variety to your walking program.

The Right Footwear

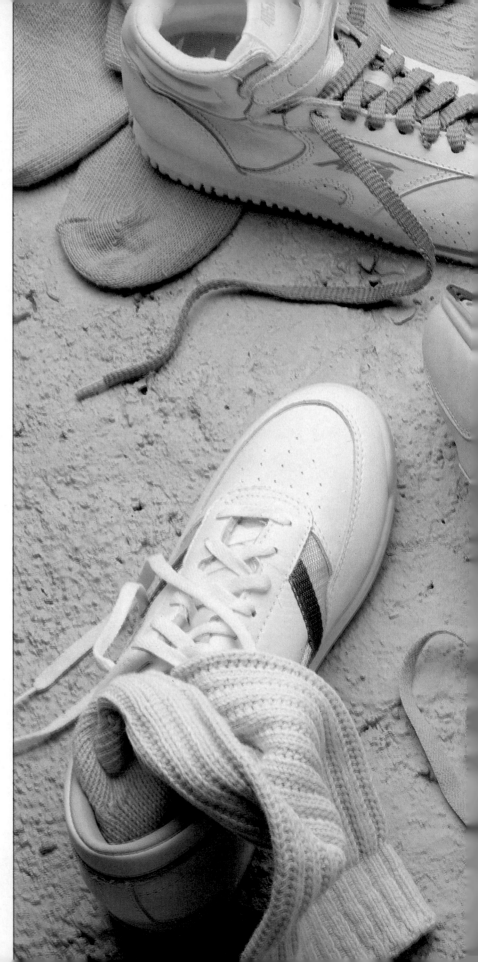

The only essential equipment for both walking and low-impact aerobic dance is an appropriate pair of shoes. Shoes for low-impact aerobic dance should feature good forefoot stability to accommodate the sideways movement that largely replaces the jumping of high-impact aerobic dance. Look for a reinforced band around the arch of the shoe and a firm heel counter, which wraps around the heel to help stabilize the foot. The shoes should also have a flexed or notched outer sole for traction and flexibility.

Some shoes with these features are designed specifically for low-impact activity, such as the shoe at bottom left. However, most standard aerobic-dance shoes are also acceptable for low-impact aerobics, although a high-top aerobic shoe, such as the one at top left, will provide extra lateral support.

Running and walking shoes are not interchangeable. The thick, shock-absorbing soles of running shoes make for unstable walking, so walking shoes feature less cushioning. They also have a rounded crash pad to absorb heelstrike. A walking shoe is more flexible than a running shoe so that the walking shoe can bend at a 45-degree angle at push-off; running shoes need flex to only 30 degrees. More grooves cut across the bottom of the walking shoe and a lower heel cushioning also contribute to greater flexibility.

Walking shoes are styled to fit various needs. There are dress walking shoes, top right; rugged walking shoes for hiking or rough terrain, bottom right; and fitness walking shoes for workouts, bottom center.

Wear socks when exercising to protect both your feet and your shoes from perspiration.

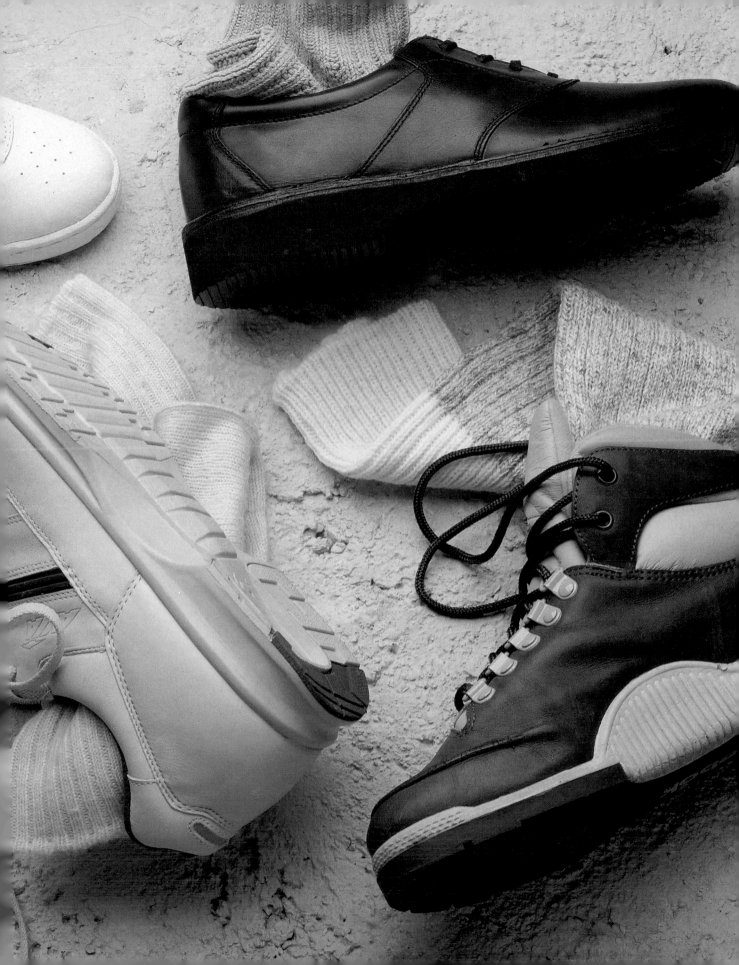

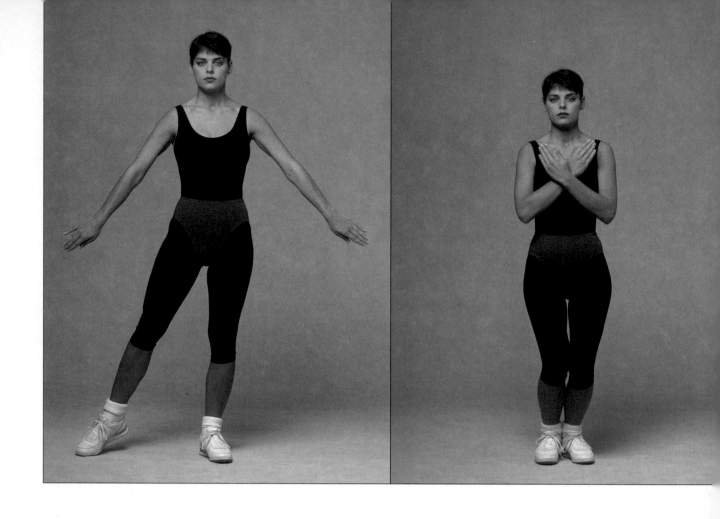

Setting Your Routine

The following routine progresses from simple sequences that focus on arm work to more complicated steps requiring you to move across the floor. Begin the routine with the warmups on these two pages and the following four; they should be sustained for at least five minutes. The cool-downs on pages 54-55 should also be done for a minimum of five minutes.

Following the warm-ups is a series of exercises in which you lunge, march, roll up on your toes and use your arms but essentially stay in one place. These precede the more complicated moving-around steps,

in which you move across the floor. Combination sequences couple the arm work of stationary sequences with the movement steps. Each sequence should be performed symmetrically, so that if you first move to your left, you should then reverse directions and repeat the exercise to your right. Repeat each sequence four times.

You will probably get the most benefit — and enjoyment — from your low-impact routine if you mix the steps in different combinations and move in different directions. You can combine sequences that use side-to-side movement with those that go forward and backward, in-

terspersed with moving-in-place steps. Be sure to vary the height of your arm movements.

As you get stronger, you will find that it becomes more difficult to achieve your target heart rate. To make your dancing more demanding, do more knee bends, take longer steps and concentrate more on moving-around sequences. You can further intensify your workout by adding hand or wrist weights. Strengthening exercises that incorporate weights into your workout are demonstrated on pages 56-61. For the greatest benefit, you should perform the routines four to five times a week.

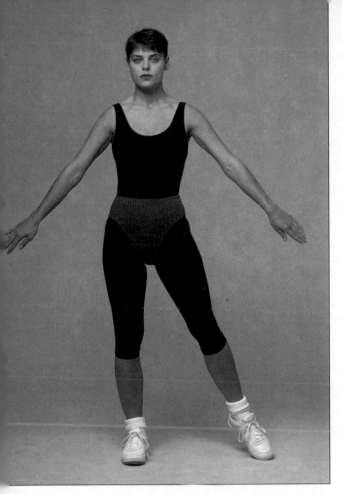

Warm-Ups/1

Stand up straight with your arms lifted slightly to the side and your right leg extended; point your toes *(far left)*. Bend your knees as you bring your feet together and swing your arms so that they cross in front of your chest *(center)*. Straighten your right leg as you repeat to your left side *(left)*.

After warming up, you can increase the intensity of the above routine by raising your arms on the extension phase. Start by bringing them to shoulder height *(left)*. When you can do this comfortably, raise them over your head *(below)*.

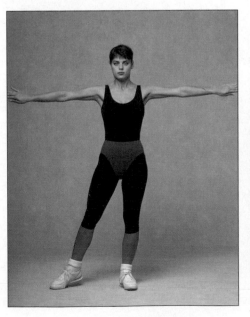

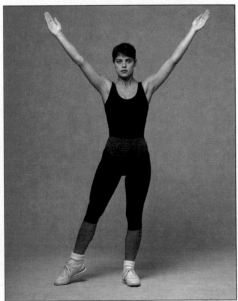

Warm-Ups/2

Stand with your feet shoulder-width apart,
toes pointed outward and arms at your
sides with your palms facing downward.
Bend your knees and push off on your
left foot, leaning to the right and lifting
your shoulder *(left)*. Bend your knees
again to recenter your weight *(center)*.
Push off to your left, lifting your right
shoulder and pointing your right foot.

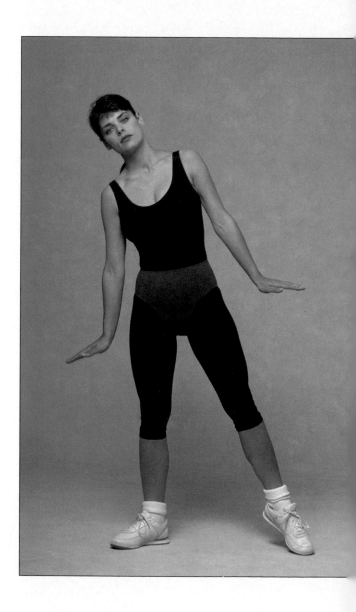

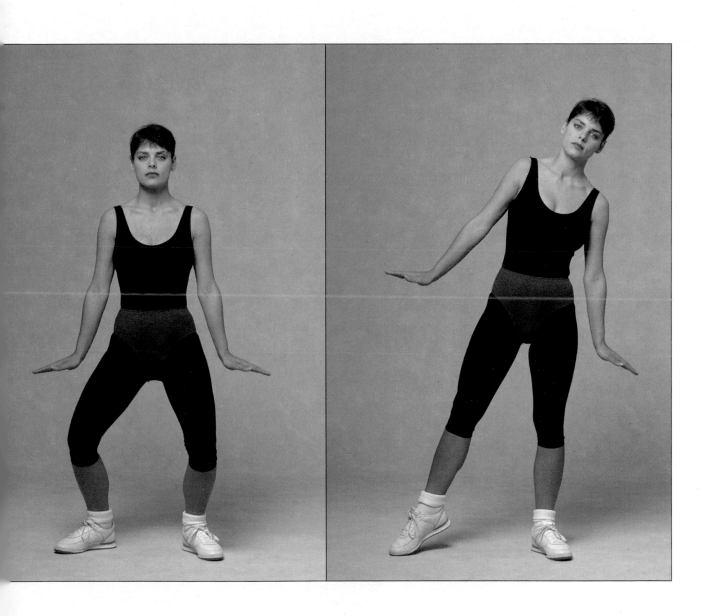

Warm-Ups/3

Stand with your feet together and knees bent. Bring your elbows back to chest height, with your palms facing forward *(right)*. Simultaneously push your hands forward and thrust your right foot out, resting it on its heel *(below)*. Return to the starting position and switch legs.

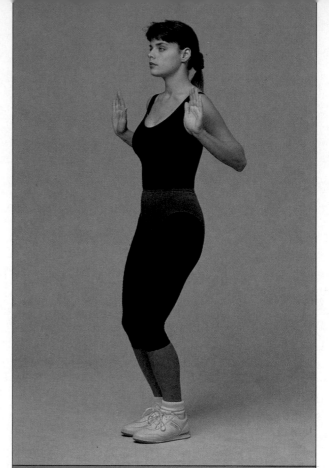

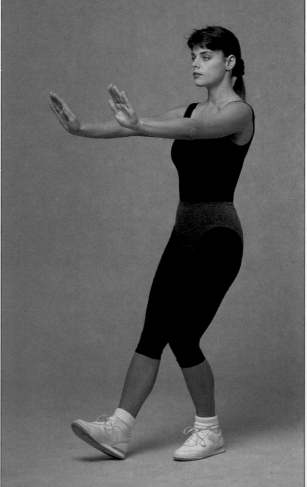

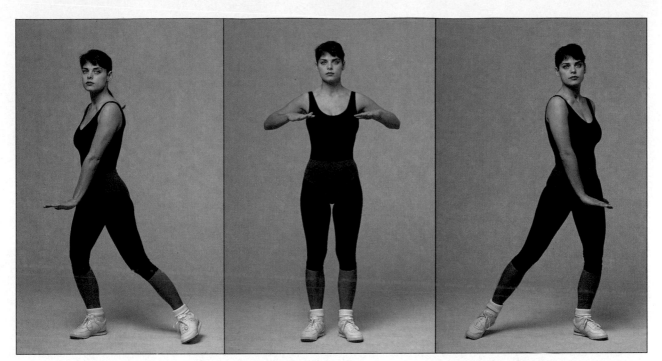

From a standing position with your arms at your sides, rotate your torso and swivel your right foot to the right as you bend your right knee. Push your hands down on either side of your body *(left)*. Bring your left foot in to your right, at the same time raising your arms in front of your chest *(center)*. Rotate to your left *(above)* and return to the center. When bending your knees, do not extend them farther than your toes.

Moving in Place/1

Stand straight with your shoulders relaxed, your abdomen contracted and your buttocks tucked under. Vigorously march in place, bringing each knee high and keeping your foot positioned directly beneath it. Land on the ball of your foot and rock to the heel on impact. Pump with your arms, holding your elbows flexed at 90-degree angles. Continue for a minute or more. You can use this as a transition step between routines.

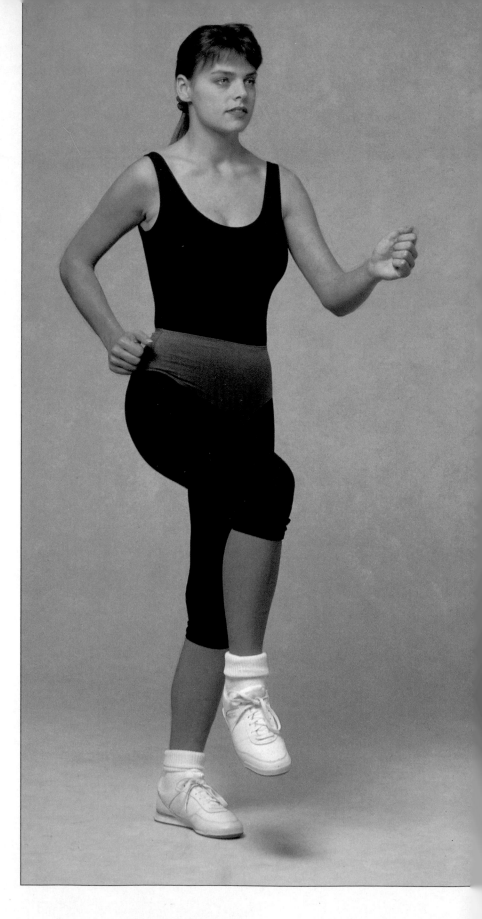

Stand with your feet together and your arms extended in front of you at shoulder height, your palms facing downward *(below).* Tilt your pelvis forward and point the toes of your right foot as you make your hands into fists and forcefully pull your arms into your sides *(bottom).* Repeat with your left leg.

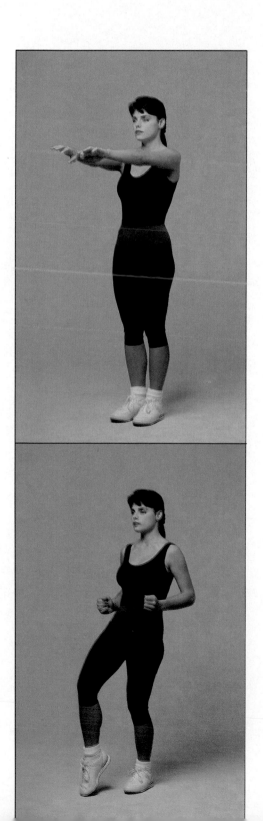

37

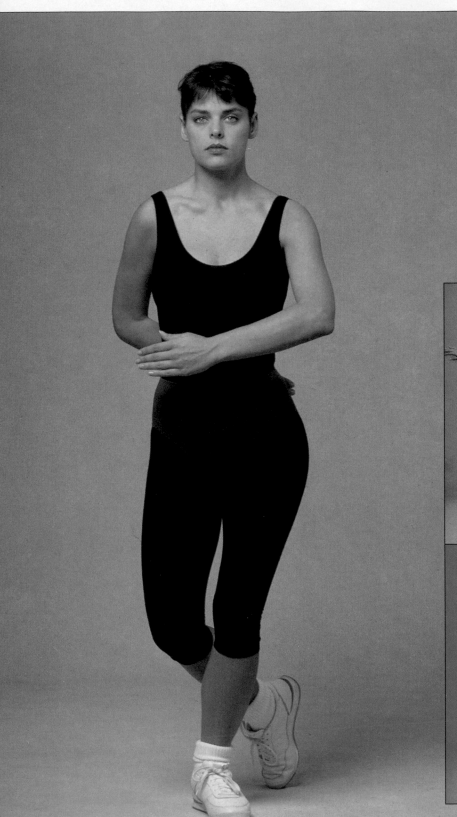

Moving in Place/2

Bend your left knee slightly as you bring your bent right leg behind you and rest on your toes. At the same time, cross your bent left arm in front of you and your bent right arm behind you *(left)*. Raise your arms to shoulder height as you extend your right leg to the side *(below)*. Shift your weight onto your right leg, dropping your heel and crossing your left leg and left arm behind you, your bent right arm in front of you *(bottom)*.

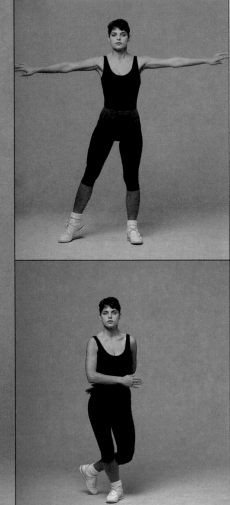

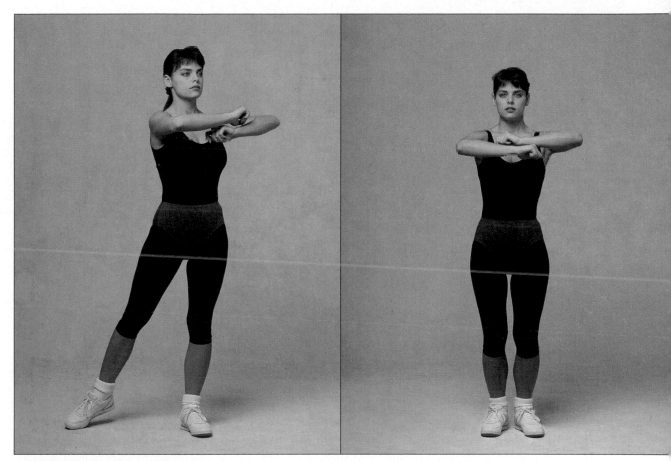

Bend your arms and hold them at
shoulder height. Roll them over each
other and rotate your torso slightly to the
left as you extend your right leg to the
side, pointing your toes *(above)*. Bend
your knees as you bring your right leg
back to your left *(right)*.

Moving in Place/3

Bend your right arm upward and touch your right elbow with your left hand. Lift your right hip as you move your right leg to the side *(below)*. Shift your weight onto your right foot and bring your left foot into your right *(center)*. Transfer your weight onto your left foot *(right)*, then back to your right.

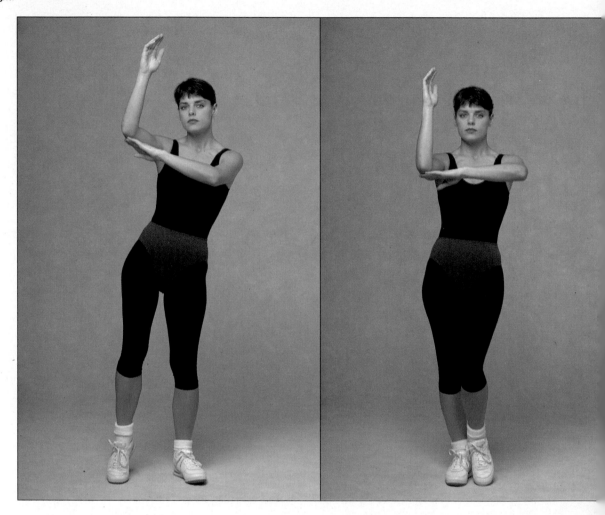

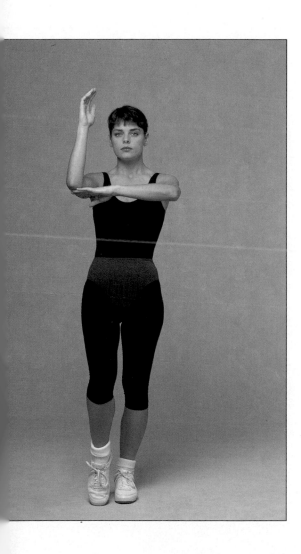

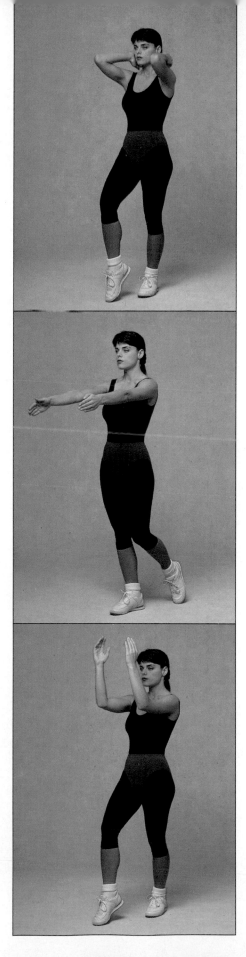

Bend your arms so that your hands are behind your shoulders and touch your right toe in front of you *(top).* Take a small step forward onto your right foot as you swing your arms forward *(center).* Touch your left toe behind you, then swing your arms back up as you step back onto your left foot and point the toe of your right foot *(right).* Leading with your right foot, march in place for seven steps; then repeat the entire sequence, beginning with your left foot.

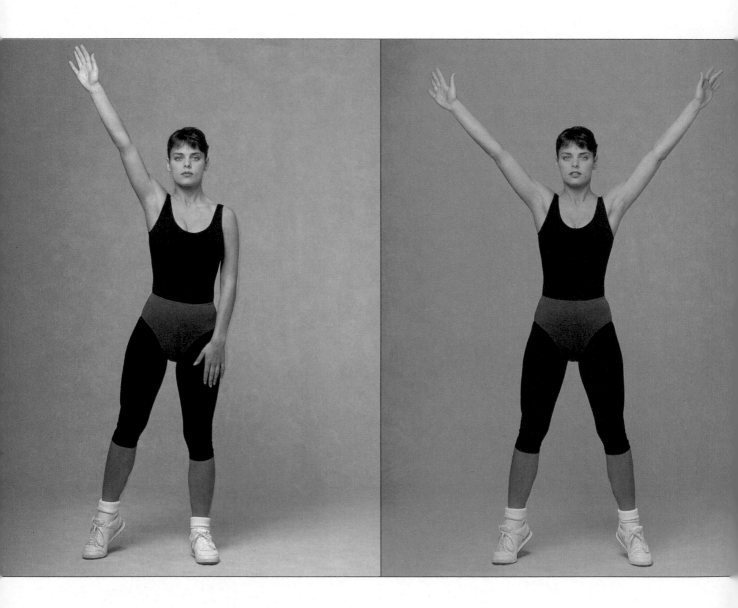

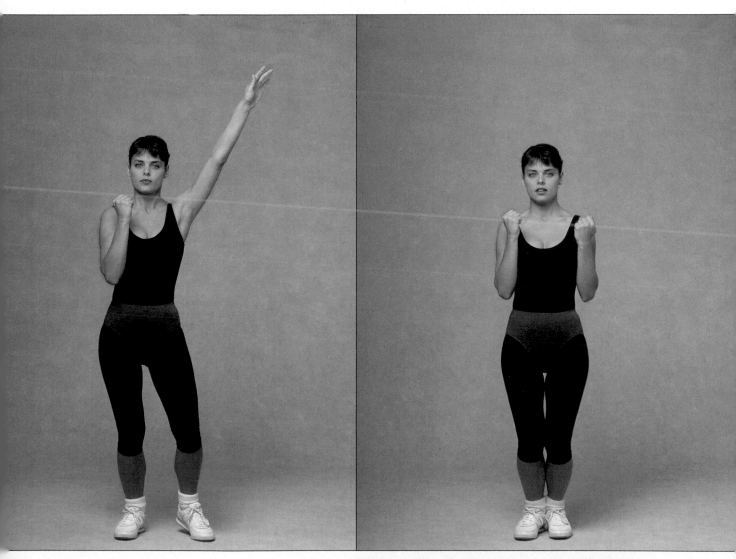

Stand up straight. Simultaneously step to the right onto the ball of your right foot and raise your right arm over your head *(far left)*. Then step to the left onto the ball of your left foot as you raise your left arm over your head *(left center)*. Bend your left knee as you step in with your right foot and bend your right elbow, pulling your arm into your chest *(right center)*. Bend both knees, bringing your left foot into your right and pulling your left arm into your chest *(above)*.

Moving Around/1

Bend your arms at the elbow, keeping your fingers straight. Step forward onto your right foot *(below)*. Rotate your arms at the elbow in a locomotive-like motion as you step forward onto your left foot *(left center)*, then forward onto your right *(right center)*. Touch your left foot to your right instep *(far right)*. Step backward onto your left foot. Continue backward with two more steps, then touch your right foot to your left instep.

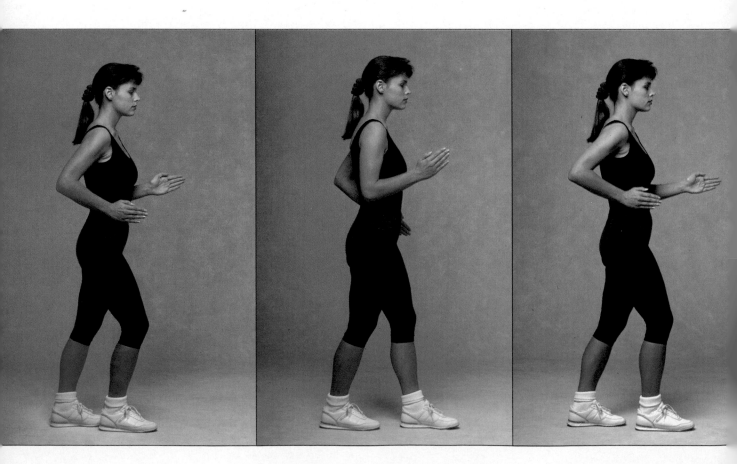

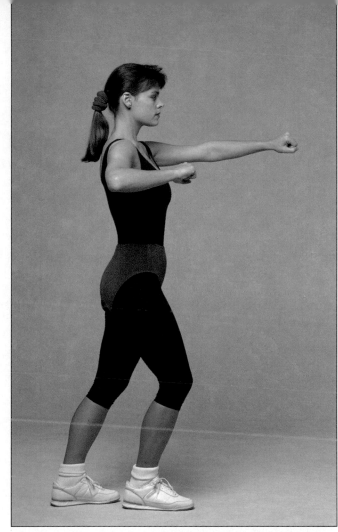

Repeat the walking sequence shown at left but bring your arms to shoulder height, using an alternate punching motion with each step.

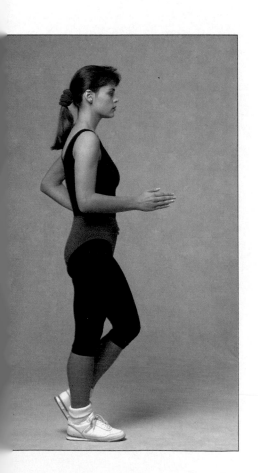

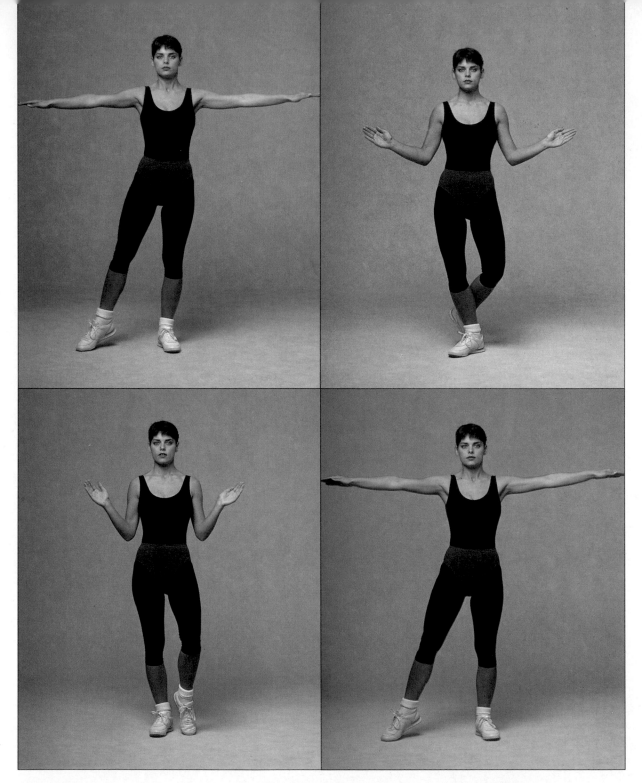

Moving Around/2

Clockwise from top left: Raise your arms to shoulder height and extend your right leg, pointing your toes. Shift your weight onto your right foot as you bend your left knee and bring your left foot behind your right, bending your elbows into your waist. Shift your weight back to your left foot and again extend your right leg to the side with your arms outstretched. Bring your elbows back into your waist as you shift onto your right foot and bring your left foot in next to your right instep.

Increase the arm work in the preceding sequence by clapping your hands over your head for the final step *(right)*. You can also cross your arms in front of you on the arm extensions, alternating the arm that is on top *(below)*.

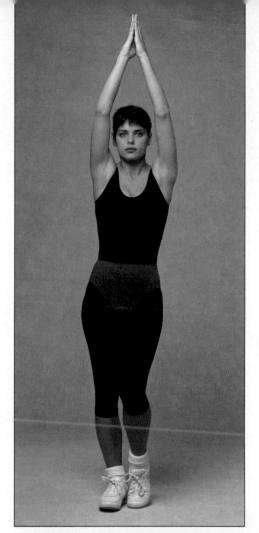

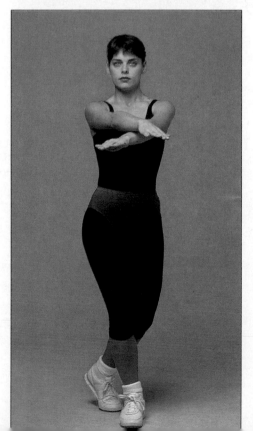

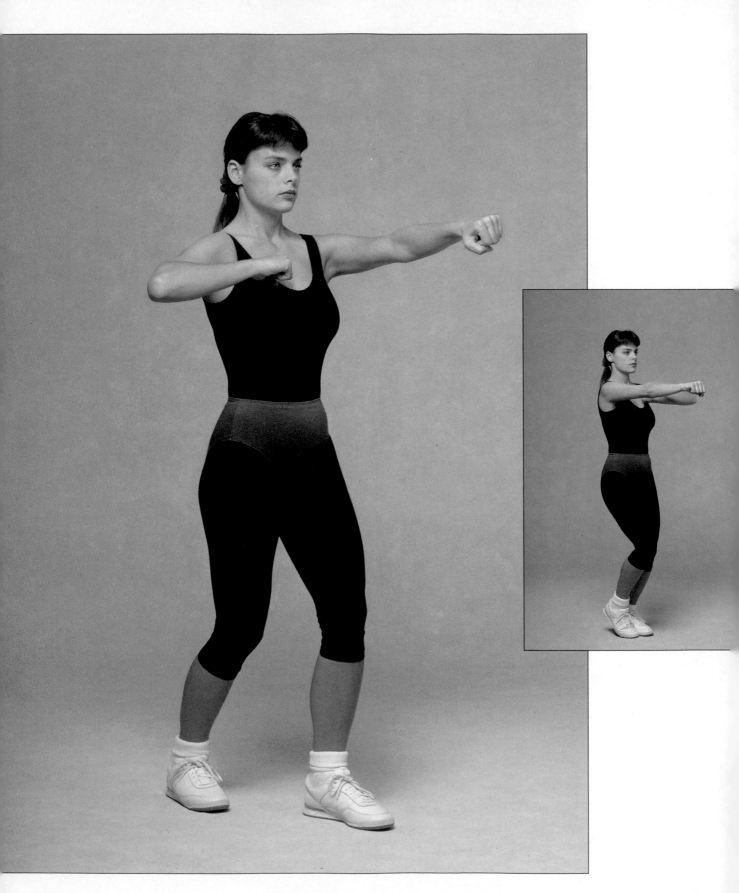

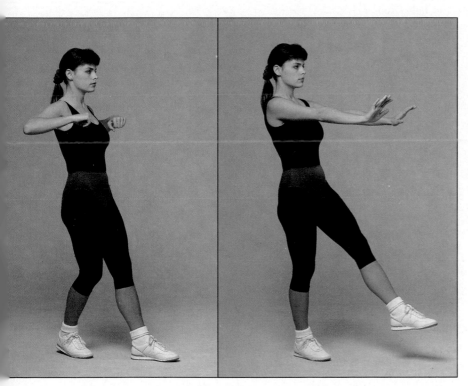

Combinations/1

Bend your elbows and bring your arms to shoulder height. Leading with your left foot, take three steps forward, punching in front of you with alternate arms *(far left)*. On the fourth step, bring your right foot forward as far as your left instep *(left center)*. Step back with your right foot as you bring your right arm back to your chest *(right center)*. Kick your left foot forward and push out with your arms *(right)*. Bring your arms back into your chest and step backward with your left foot. Kick your right foot forward, extending your arms. Go back two more steps, kick, then lower your right foot next to your left.

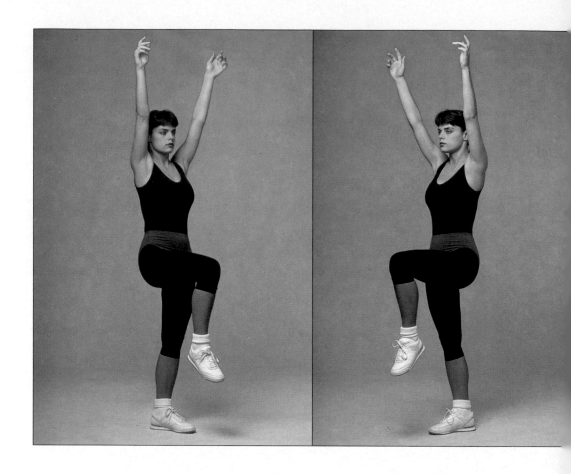

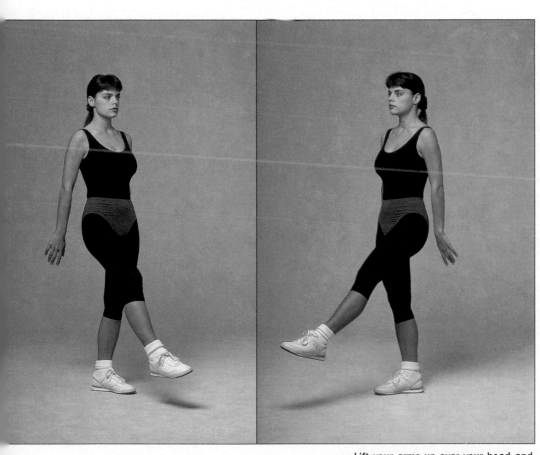

Lift your arms up over your head and, turning to your left, bring your bent right leg up to hip height *(far left)*. Bend your elbows and drop your arms and leg; repeat, then pivot to your right and lift your arms upward again, this time lifting your left knee *(center left)*. Drop your leg and arms, repeat, then pivot back to your left, kicking your right foot forward and pushing back with your arms *(center right)*. Bring your arms and leg back, then repeat once. Pivot to your right and kick with your left leg twice *(above)*.

Combinations/3

Swing your arms and hips to the right as you lean into your right hip *(below)*, then swing to the left; repeat. On the final swing, bring your left foot behind your right *(center)*. Rise onto the toes of your left foot and step to the right with your right leg, swinging your arms back to the right. Touch the ball of your left foot to your right instep, then extend your leg back to the left as you clap your hands overhead *(right)*.

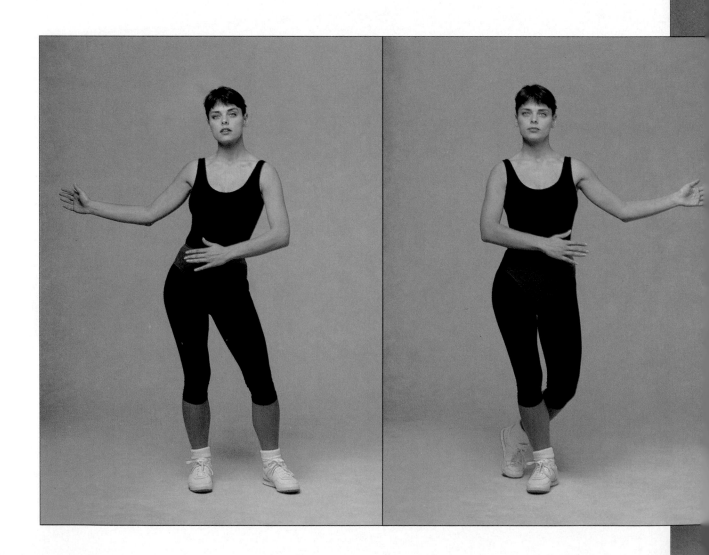

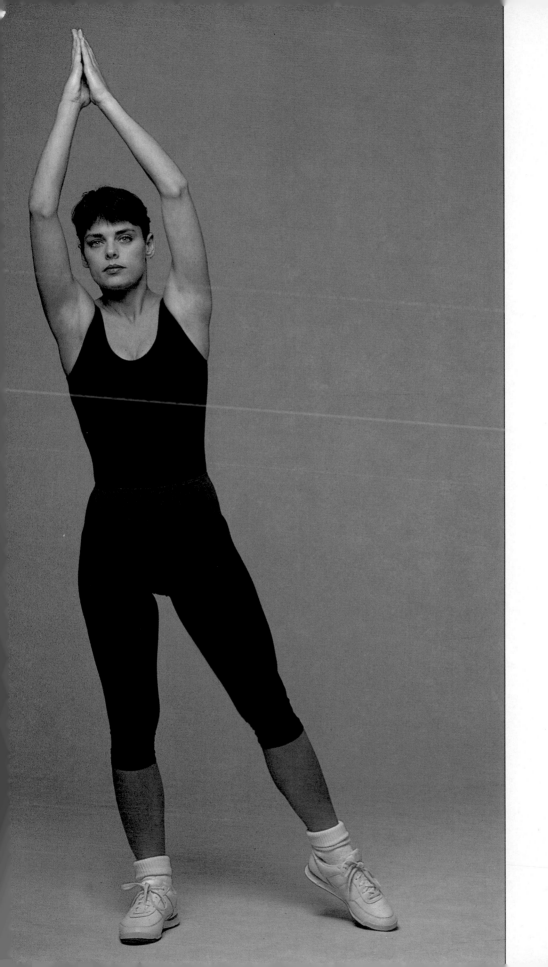

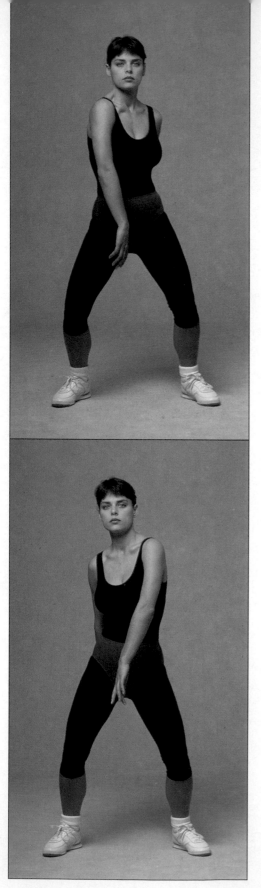

Cool-Downs

Stand with your feet about shoulder-width apart, your toes pointing outward. Bend your knees slightly as you rotate your right arm at the shoulder, bringing it downward in a crawl-like swimming motion *(left)*. Straighten your legs and bring your right shoulder back, then flex your knees again as you repeat with your left arm *(below)*.

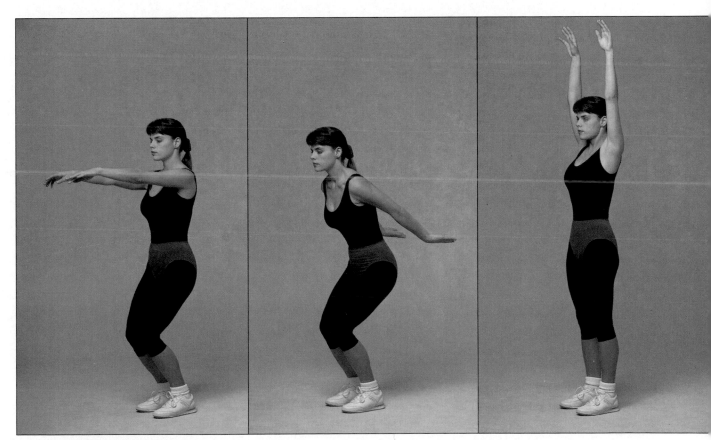

From a standing position, raise your arms
in front of you at shoulder level and bend
your knees *(above)*. Start to swing your
arms down and straighten your knees.
Bring your arms behind you, bending your
knees again *(center)*, then swing your
arms up toward the ceiling. Straighten
your body as you extend your arms
overhead *(right)*.

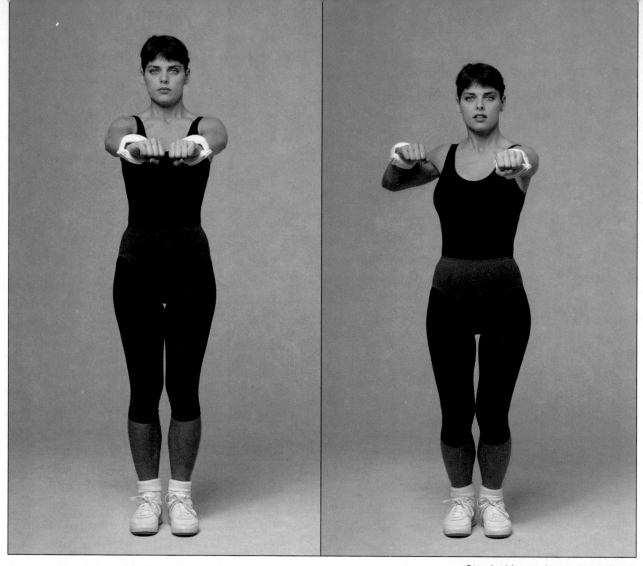

Stand with your knees bent slightly and your arms raised to shoulder level *(above left)*. Bend your knees, pulling your bent right arm backward so your fist is about level with your shoulder *(above)*. Straighten your legs as you return to the starting position, then repeat with your left arm.

Adding Weights/1

Weights help to intensify an aerobic dance program, but they should only be incorporated once you can easily perform your usual routine without reaching your target heart rate. An indication of the right time to add weights is when you can perform 16 repetitions of the same step without becoming fatigued. This is a sign that your body has adapted to a higher level of fitness. Adding additional weights will place more de-

mands on your cardiovascular system, boosting your heart rate back into its target range.

Begin with the lightest hand weights, usually a half-pound per hand. (Because of the stress they add to the shin, the Achilles tendon and the back, ankle weights are not recommended during aerobic exercise.) As your body adapts to this new load, you can increase the weights by half-pound intervals. Do not use weights heavier than three

pounds each when performing low-impact aerobics.

Hold the weights firmly but not tightly — the isometric pressure of tight gripping can impair blood flow in the arms and thus raise blood pressure. If you develop muscle pain or joint soreness, stop using weights until the pain disappears. Consult your physician if the pain persists. When you are ready to take up weights again, begin with a light load, and increase it gradually.

Stand with your knees slightly bent and your arms at your sides with your elbows bent *(right)*. Move both arms behind you as far as possible, keeping your elbows bent *(center).* Return to the starting position.

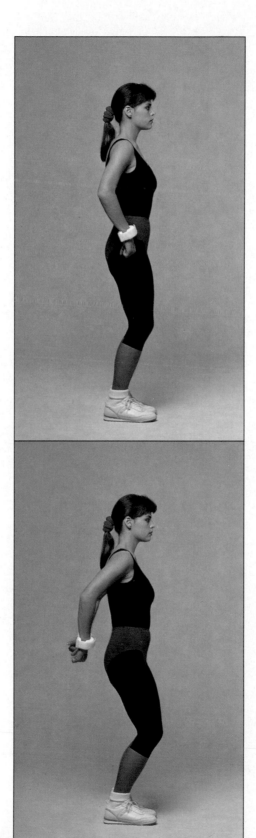

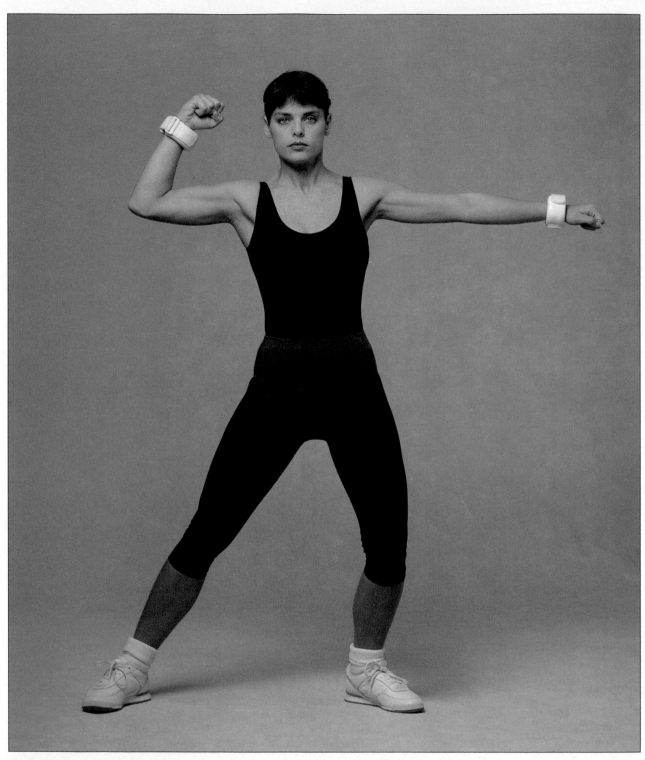

Stand with your legs shoulder-width apart and your arms outstretched at shoulder height. Lunge to the left as you extend your left arm and bend your right elbow (above).

Adding Weights/2

From a standing position with your arms at your sides, step to your right, so your feet are shoulder-width apart and your knees are bent. Your arms should be at shoulder height with your elbows flexed *(below left)*. Simultaneously pull your elbows into your sides and bring your right foot back to center *(center)*. Repeat the arm motion as you step to your left. Vary the motion by raising your arms over your head when you step in *(below)*, then pulling them down to shoulder height when you step out. Keep your elbows bent when you raise your arms over your head.

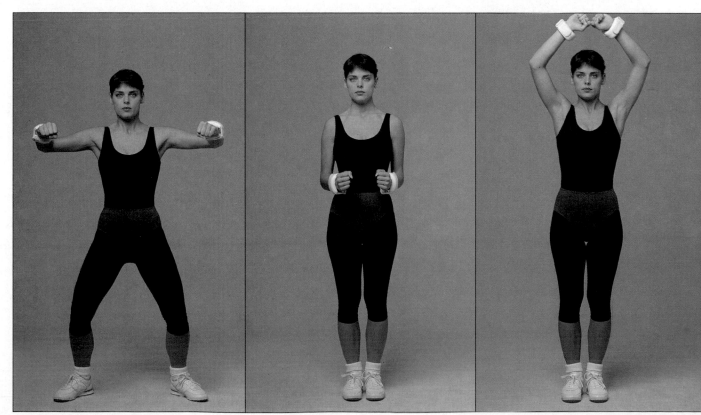

Adding Weights/3

Raise your bent arms to shoulder height. As you lift your left knee to hip level *(right)*, pull your arms down to touch slightly under your bent knee *(below)*, then bring the arms back up as you put your left leg down and raise your right. Keep your back straight.

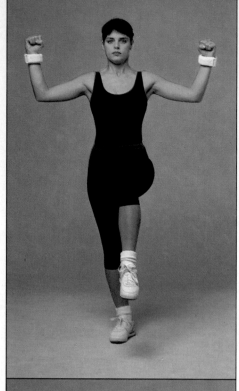

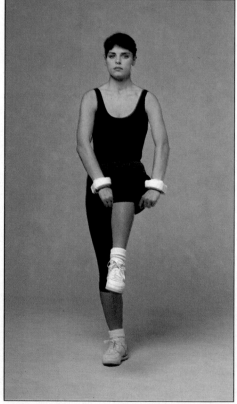

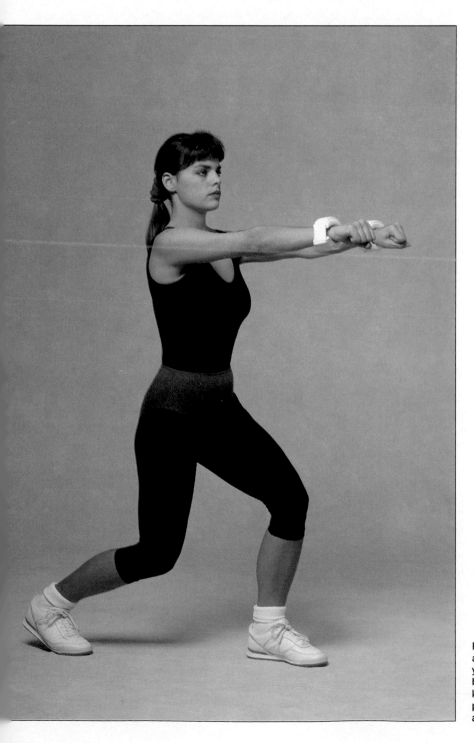

From a standing position, extend your
arms directly in front of you. Push off on
your left foot to lunge backward onto the
ball of your right foot. Keep your back
knee bent *(left)*. Return to the starting
position by pushing off your back foot
and bringing you arms into your chest.

61

Your Walking Program

When performed aerobically, walking provides important cardiovascular benefits comparable to those associated with more strenuous aerobic exercise such as running and cycling. Numerous studies have confirmed that walking can improve circulation and lung capacity.

To achieve aerobic benefits from walking or any other activity, you need to exercise vigorously enough to attain your target heart rate, then sustain it for at least 20 minutes. Researchers have found that most individuals are able to reach their target heart rates at walking speeds of between three and a half and four and a half miles an hour. Changing your pace from strolling (at three miles an hour or slower) to striding (at four miles an hour or faster) increases your energy expenditure — as measured in calories — by up to a third, as the chart opposite shows. To determine your walking pace, see the chart at the bottom of the opposite page.

When you walk at a moderate pace, your level of exertion approaches that of swimming, as the chart below shows. If you intensify your walking workout, as demonstrated on pages 66-67, your energy output will approximate that of slow running; however, your body will not be at risk for the physical stresses that contribute to the high rate of running injuries. The biomechanical aspects of walking are explained on pages 64-65. Retro walking, a way to work your muscles differently and add variety to your walking regimen, is described on pages 68-69.

WALKING VS. OTHER ACTIVITIES

Activity	Calories
Slow running (5.5 mph)	
Recreational tennis, singles	
Swimming, slow crawl	
Leisure cycling (7 mph)	
Uphill walking, 10% incline (3 mph)	
Brisk walking (5 mph)	
Walking with a 15-pound backpack (4 mph)	
Moderate walking (3 mph)	

100   200   300   400   500

Calories

This chart compares the number of calories expended by a 150-pound person during one hour of various activities. Add 10 percent for every 15 pounds over this weight; subtract 10 percent for every 15 pounds under.

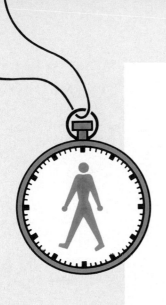

CALORIES BURNED BY WALKING FOR ONE HOUR

MPH	WEIGHT					
	100	120	140	160	180	200
3.0	180	220	260	300	340	380
3.5	220	260	300	340	380	420
4.0	250	300	350	400	450	500
4.5	280	340	400	460	520	580
5.0	320	380	450	530	610	690

WALKING SPEED CONVERSION TABLE

Steps per minute		Minutes per mile		Miles per hour
70		30		2
90		24		2.5
105		20		3
120		17		3.5
140		15		4
160		13		4.5
175		12		5
190		11		5.5
210+		<10		>6

To estimate your walking speed, count how many steps you take per minute and compare the results with this table. This rate is based on an average stride (2.5 feet long); stride length will vary from person to person.

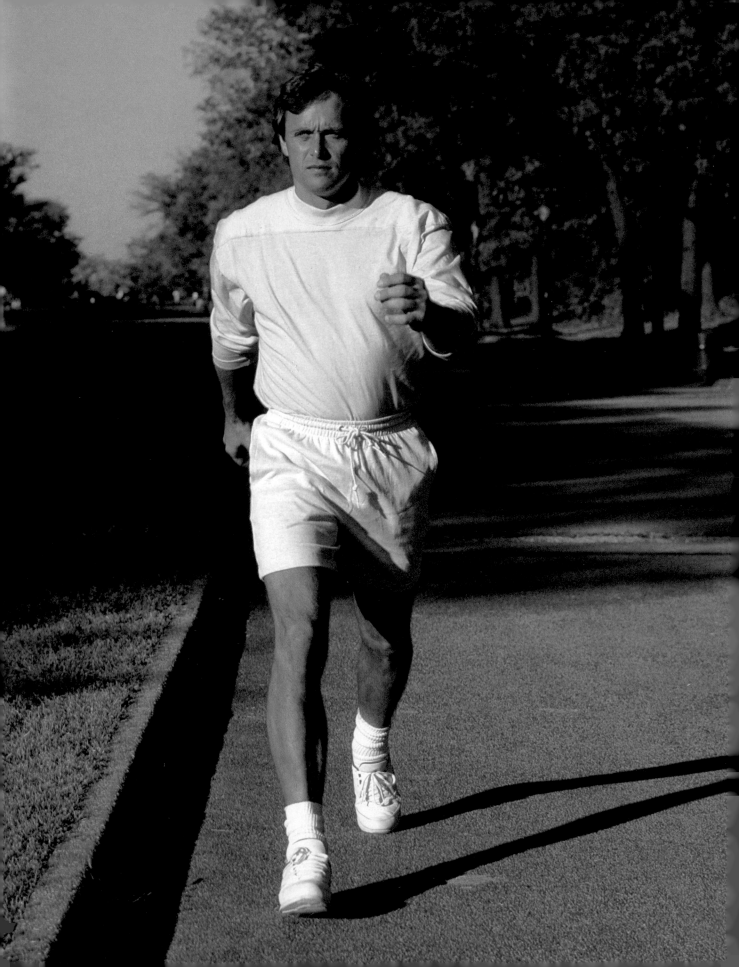

Biomechanics of Walking

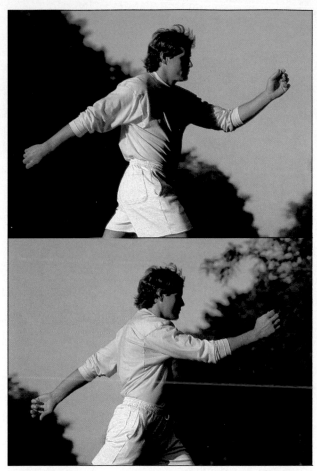

For fitness walking, your forward arm should be bent at about a 90-degree angle, with your fists clenched loosely *(top)*. The arm behind you should just brush your side as it pumps forward and the other arm swings backward *(above)*.

Walking conditions the whole body, but particularly the legs. The flexing of your foot when it lands strengthens the shins, while pushing off at the heel strengthens the calf muscles and the hamstrings along the back of the leg. Likewise, extending the leg in the forward stride tones the quadriceps in the front of the thigh; the hip flexors and buttocks muscles are worked by lengthening your stride. In addition, fitness walking conditions the abdominals, and swinging the arms works the arm and shoulder muscles.

Proper posture is important to effective walking: Stand straight with your shoulders back but relaxed. Your arms should move in opposition to your legs *(opposite)*. Plant your feet almost in front of each other, as if you were walking along an imaginary line.

Do some simple stretching exercises both before and after your workout to warm up and cool down.

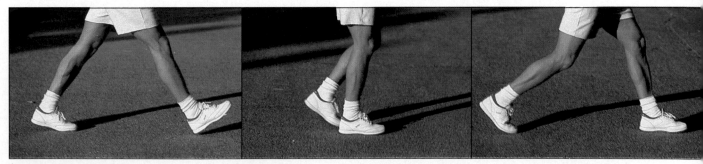

On impact, plant your foot so that your heel lands first at about a 90-degree angle to your leg and a 45-degree angle to the ground *(above)*. Rock forward as your trailing foot begins to lift off the ground *(center)*. Roll forward on your back foot to push off the ground with your toes and complete the stride *(right)*.

Reaching for Higher Intensity

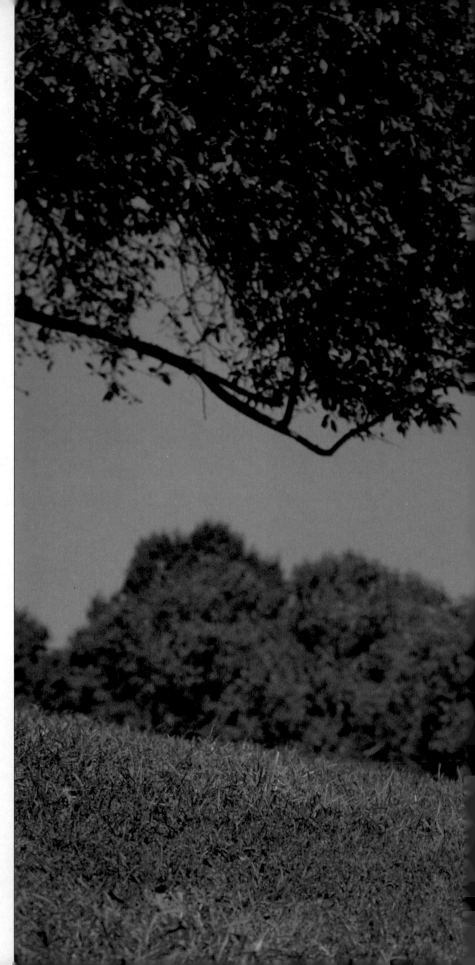

As your walking program progresses, your cardiovascular system will become more efficient, so that, even when you are walking as fast as you comfortably can, you will have difficulty reaching your target heart rate. This is an indication that you need to intensify your walking.

One of the best ways to increase the effort and the benefits of walking is to incorporate hill work *(right)*. Walking up a 10 percent incline can almost double the energy costs of walking the same distance on level ground; steeper grades increase the effort further. Lean forward slightly when walking uphill and swing your arms vigorously.

Walking downhill requires more effort than walking on level ground but less effort than walking uphill. The extra work of downhill walking is due to the exertion required to brake your acceleration.

Carrying weights as you walk is another effective way of making your workout more demanding. You will receive the greatest benefit from combining hand weights with vigorous arm swings *(see chart page 16)*. This combination will result in an energy expenditure comparable to slow jogging. (If you have any back problems, you should probably avoid using hand weights.) Begin with one-pound weights and work up to three pounds.

A final way to add both variety and intensity to your walking is to vary the terrain. When you walk on a beach, the resistance offered by sand increases energy output by almost a third. Hiking is even more strenuous; you may expend 50 percent more energy walking on a trail than you would on a paved road.

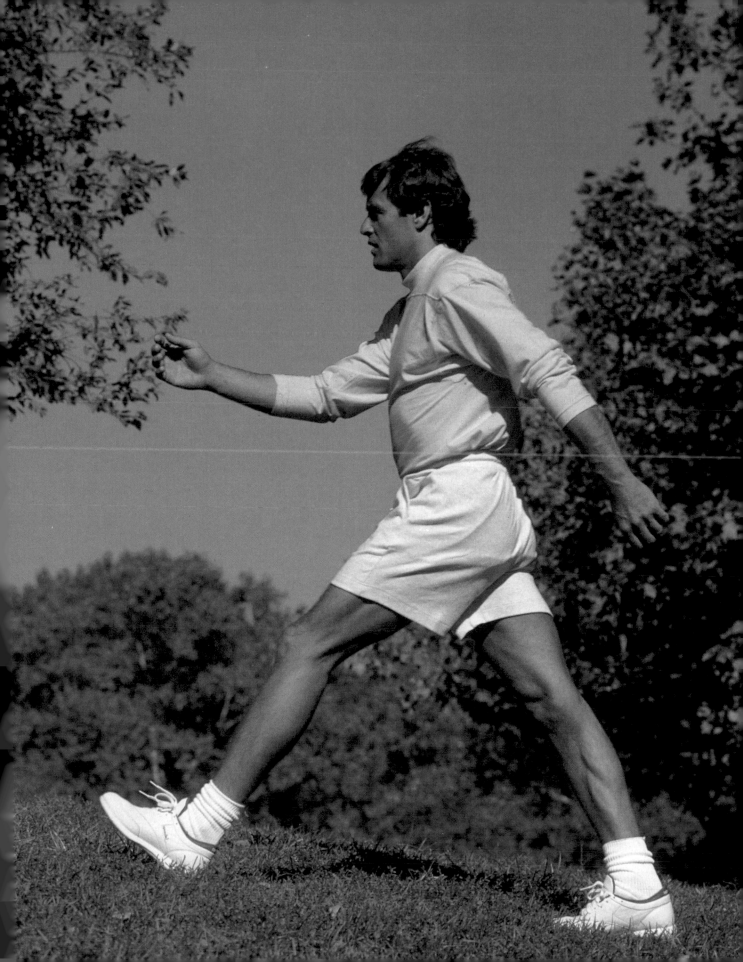

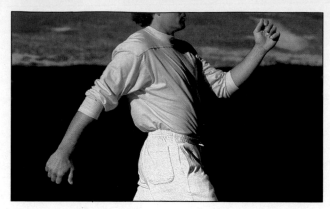

Pump your arms as you do in forward walking. Extend your arms slightly to the sides to aid in balance.

Retro Walking

Retro, or backward, movement is commonly used in many sports, such as soccer, basketball and tennis. Recently it has gained acceptance as a means of injury rehabilitation. It also aids in achieving muscle balance by strengthening opposing muscles.

Studies have shown that retro walking is not merely the mirror image of forward walking; indeed, there are very distinct biomechanical differences in body position and the use of the legs. The greatest difference is in the action of the knee joint. Retro walking affords the knee an increased range of motion, which results in a greater stretch of the hamstrings. The range of motion required in the hip joint is decreased in retro walking, which places less stress on the hip muscles. In addition, preliminary studies indicate that the energy expenditure of backward movement is greater than that of forward movement.

You can incorporate up to a quarter mile of retro walking into your walking workout; this is sufficient to give you its unique benefits. Bear in mind that retro walking does have a drawback — the danger of bumping into something or falling. You should never retro walk on a street. A track is ideal, but any smooth surface without traffic will do. Periodically check to see what is behind you by looking over your shoulder — alternate shoulders to prevent neck cramping — or walk with a partner who moves forward as you walk backward.

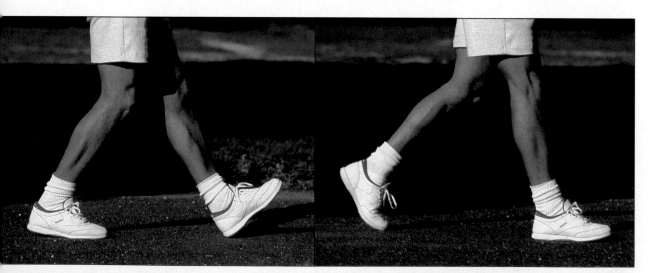

In retro walking, the push-off phase is accomplished with the heel of your forward foot (left). The leg then swings back and lands on the forefoot (above).

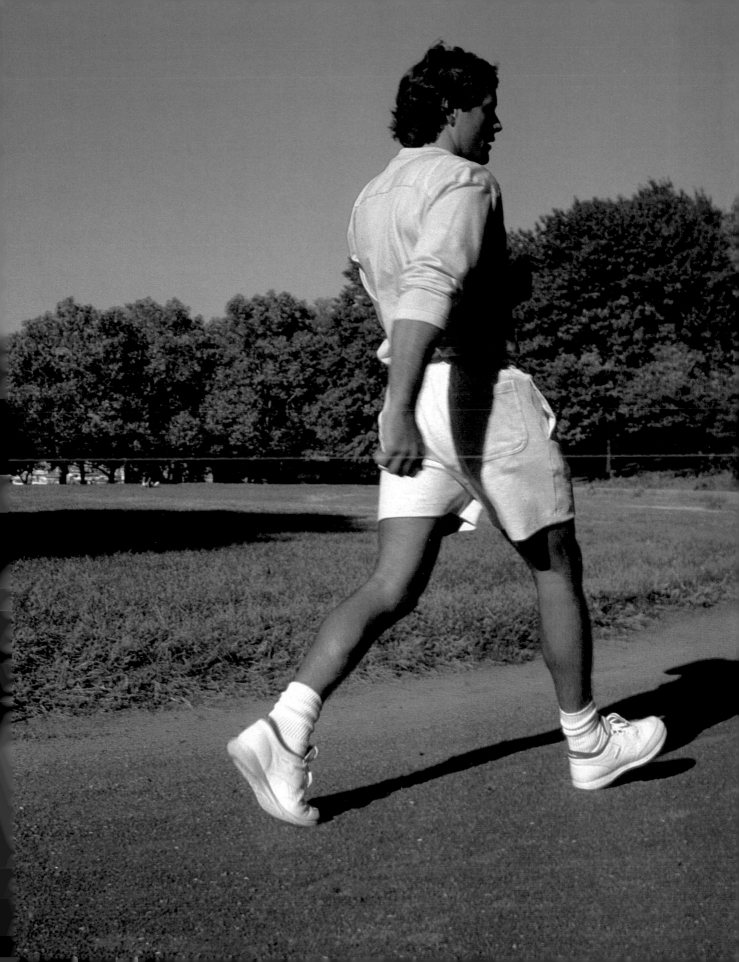

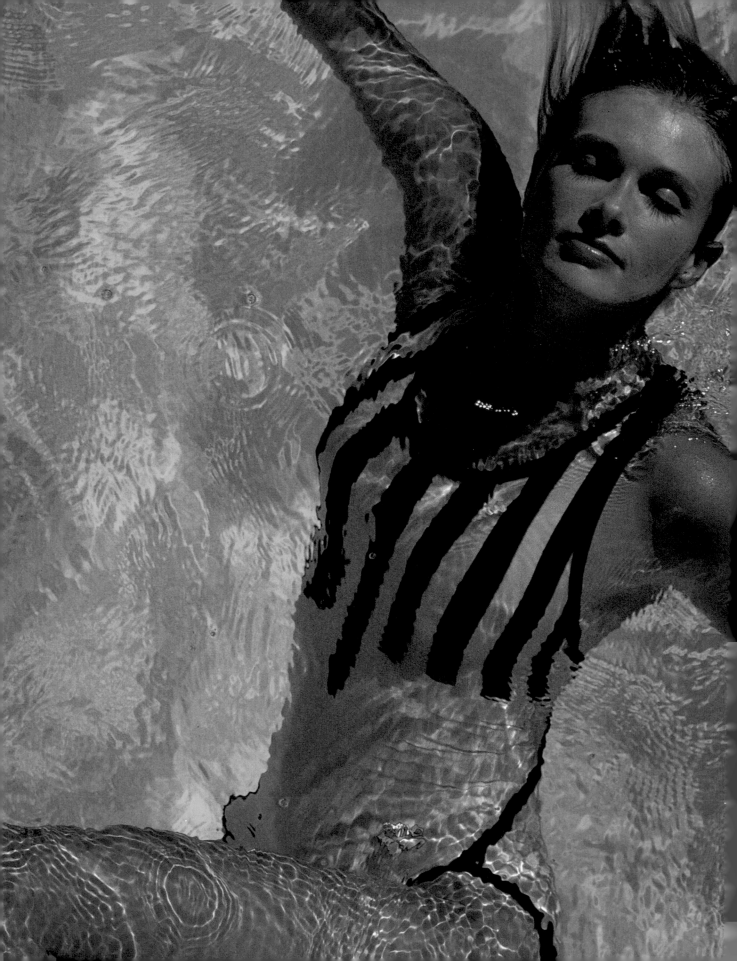

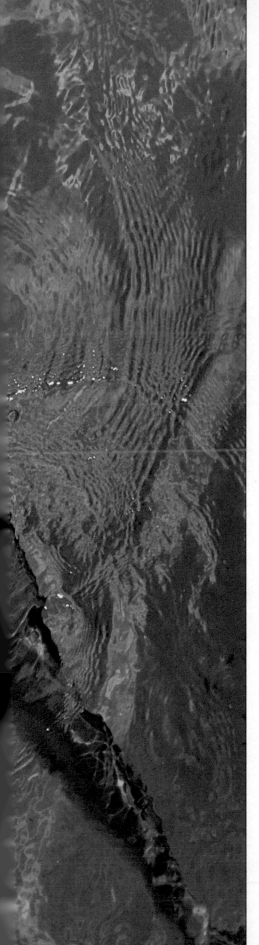

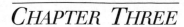

CHAPTER THREE

Water Workouts

*Versatile routines in a virtually
stress-free environment*

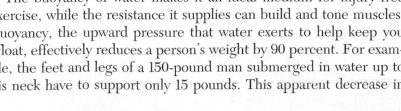

S wimming is often considered an ideal exercise because of its superlative conditioning benefits coupled with low rates of injury. But nonswimming water workouts can incorporate many of these benefits, and even work some additional muscles not used in swimming. A carefully designed water exercise regimen can be a comprehensive program that targets all four major areas of fitness: flexibility, coordination, strength and endurance. And anyone who has access to an indoor pool can compensate for having to curtail other seasonal exercises.

The buoyancy of water makes it an ideal medium for injury-free exercise, while the resistance it supplies can build and tone muscles. Buoyancy, the upward pressure that water exerts to help keep you afloat, effectively reduces a person's weight by 90 percent. For example, the feet and legs of a 150-pound man submerged in water up to his neck have to support only 15 pounds. This apparent decrease in

71

weight means that less stress is placed on the joints and ligaments. In fact, an impetus for the development of water workouts has been the success of hydrotherapy, or rehabilitation in water following injury, which often returns damaged joints and muscles to full usage and range of motion more quickly than other types of physical therapy.

The buoyancy of water also makes it an especially good exercise environment for handicapped, overweight or pregnant individuals for whom weight-bearing exercise is difficult. But water workouts can also benefit anyone who exercises, from beginners to professional athletes. Indeed, many coaches are now incorporating pool workouts into their teams' training programs. In an effort to cut back on the injuries sustained in competitive cross-country running, the coach of Yale University's cross-country team recently eliminated one of the team's two daily workouts on land and substituted running in deep water. Although the runners' weekly mileage dropped from 60 to 70 miles to between 45 and 50 miles, the team had a championship — and virtually injury-free — season. Overall, water workouts reduced stress injuries by 90 percent.

Water running is one of many pool exercises that are simply land exercises performed in water. Research has shown that such exercises translated into a water medium can provide benefits to the heart, lungs and circulation comparable to the same exercises done on land. One university study compared the cardiovascular effects of water and land running in 16 runners. Half the group trained as usual, while the rest ran in deep water, using flotation devices to maintain an upright posture. The water runners showed no significant decrease in VO_2max, an important gauge of cardiovascular fitness that measures the ability to take in and use oxygen.

The resistance of water, which is about 800 times heavier than air, makes exercising in it very effective for muscle development; this resistance means that an exercise performed in the water requires more effort than the same exercise done on land. For example, if you run an eight-minute mile on dry land, it will take you 30 minutes to run the same distance in waist-high water. And the deeper the water, the more difficult the exercise. One study of walking in water found that water depth was a significant factor in the metabolic costs of the activity. Using a submerged treadmill, researchers measured oxygen consumption in 11 subjects at a range of walking speeds and at varying water depths. Walkers at all water depths showed significantly higher VO_2max than those walking on land. Interestingly, another study found that the metabolic costs of water walking are more than twice as great as land walking, while the energy uptakes of both land and water running are essentially the same. Researchers attribute this to the difficulty of maintaining proper running form in the water.

Water resistance is also exerted evenly in all directions. This constant pressure makes water ideal for strengthening exercises because it works opposing muscle groups equally. By contrast, most weight-training is based on resistance to gravity and works one muscle group

Getting Started

◆ One important factor in effective water workouts is your choice of swimming pool. Try to find one with a bottom that slopes gradually, allowing you to stand in water up to your waist at one point, and your shoulders at another. A gutter or swim trough around the perimeter will allow you to perform certain exercises that require gripping an edge or hoisting yourself out of the water. For some exercises, grasping the top rung of a pool ladder will suffice.

◆ Aquatic equipment can enhance or intensify your workout. Flotation vests provide support for water running and walking; they also allow you to work out in deep water if you are a nonswimmer. Kickboards let you practice your swim kicks. Hand paddles provide extra resistance for arm work; fins do the same for your legs.

◆ The pool and its environs should be well maintained. Although cloudy pool water does not necessarily imply that upkeep is substandard, the proper chemical balance is important for your health. Check with an attendant if you have any doubts. As a rule, if the water is clear enough so that you can see the drain at the deep end, the pool is sufficiently clean.

◆ Good posture is essential for the effective performance of many of the water workouts demonstrated in this chapter. If you keep your abdomen and buttocks muscles tucked in as you exercise, you will avoid the pressure on lower back muscles that overarching your back can cause. Be sure that you remain relaxed as you go through each exercise sequence.

at a time, leaving open the possibility that opposing muscle groups will not get equivalent workouts.

The resistance of water can be controlled: The more you push against it, the more it will resist. Adjusting the speed at which you perform a particular motion will vary the resistance and thus your energy expenditure. Furthermore, the constant resistance encountered in water means that virtually any type of exercise includes a strengthening element. For example, the leg stretches on pages 82-83 are basically flexibility exercises, but because of the water resistance, these exercises also strengthen the muscles of the legs.

Because almost all the exercises in this chapter can be performed while standing in the water, you need not be a swimmer to get the benefits of these workouts. However, the naturally low-impact benefits of swimming can intensify your workout. A number of the following exercises isolate various swimming motions — the arm movement used in the breaststroke or the leg motion in the flutter kick, for example. Nonswimmers can perform these exercises at the side of the pool or holding onto a kickboard to attain some of the specific muscular and cardiovascular benefits of swimming. Of course, if you enjoy swimming, you are encouraged to add this activity to your low-impact exercise regimen.

A Complete Routine

The comprehensive workout on the following 14 pages is divided into three sections: strengtheners, stretches for flexibility and aerobics. The swimming movements on pages 90-95 enhance coordination, thus rounding out a fitness program.

Work out in a pool whose temperature is between 80 and 84 degrees F. You may be more comfortable performing routines that call for relatively high levels of exertion in water between 78 and 82 degrees F.

The natural cooling effect of water coupled with its buoyancy means that you might not be fully aware of the workload your muscles are subjected to, but a water workout can be as intense as any land-based regimen. Therefore, you should devote at least five minutes to the warm-ups on these two pages to prepare your muscles for exertion; after your workout, spend at least five minutes on cool-downs (*pages 96-97*). Perform each of the following exercises 10 times or for one minute if it is a continuous activity like running. Increase these repetitions gradually as you become more conditioned. Work toward 20-30 repetitions or three to five minutes of continuous activity.

Also, be sure to drink water before and after you exercise in a pool: Even though you may not realize it, you perspire when you exercise in water, particularly during an aerobic workout.

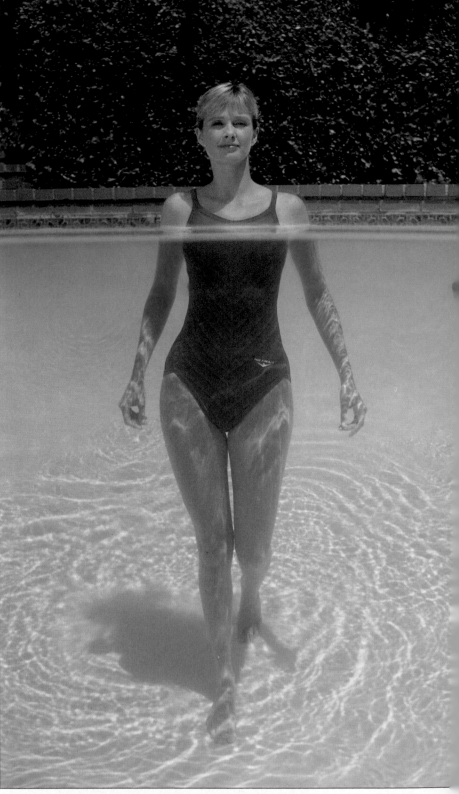

Stand in chest-high water. Walk around the pool, keeping the same form you would use if you were walking on land: Hold your head high and do not lean too far forward. Swing your arms as you alternate legs.

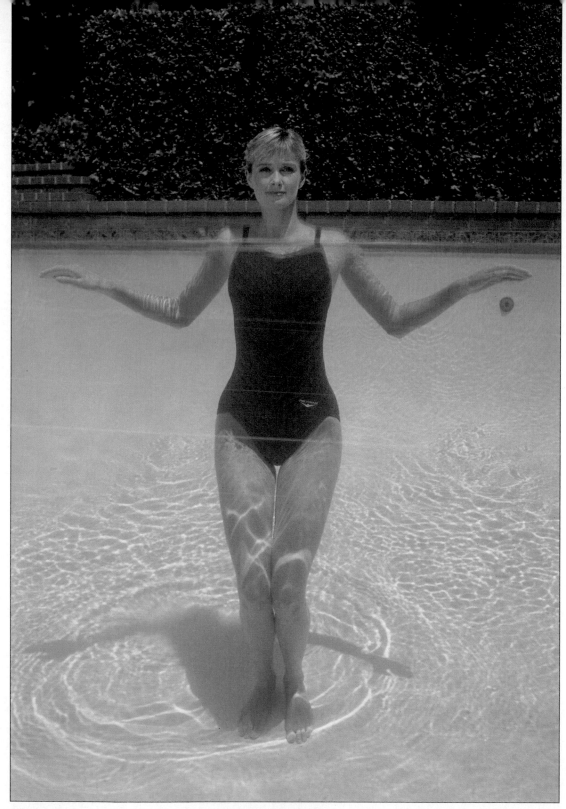

Stand erect in chest-high water with your arms at your sides. Keeping your back straight, flex your knees and lower yourself until the water is shoulder level. Bend your elbows and extend your arms for support. Bob.

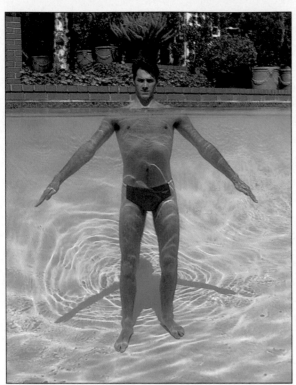

Strengtheners/1

Stand in water to your neck with your feet spread. Extend your arms from your sides at about a 45-degree angle and rotate them in small circles *(top left)*. Then raise your arms to shoulder height and rotate them in small circles *(bottom left)*.

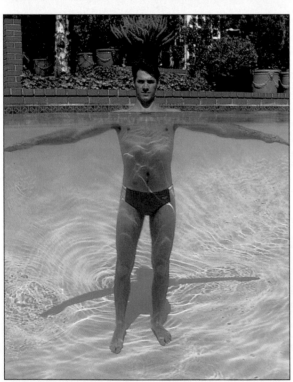

Stand at arm's length from the edge of the pool in chest-high water. Spread your feet slightly and grasp the edge *(opposite)*. Keep your back straight as you bend your arms and lean inward to bring your chin next to the edge *(inset left)*. Push out to return to the original position, then push off on your feet, straightening your arms to hold you next to the pool with your upper body out of the water *(inset right)*.

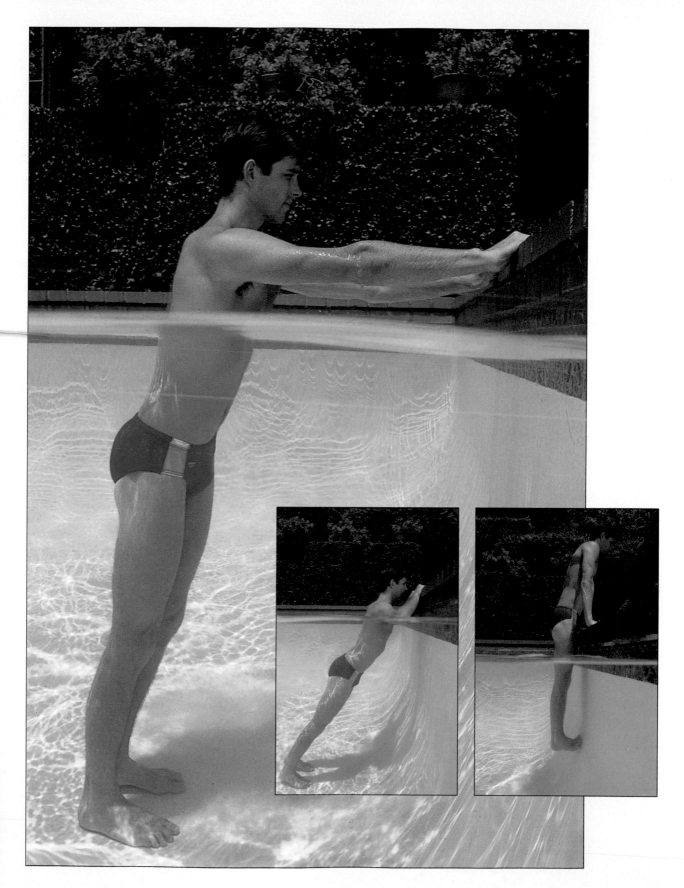

Strengtheners/2

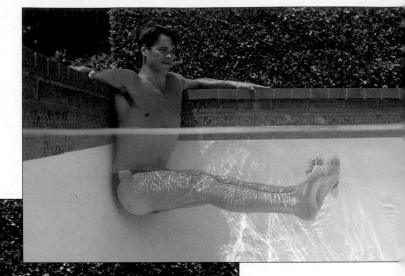

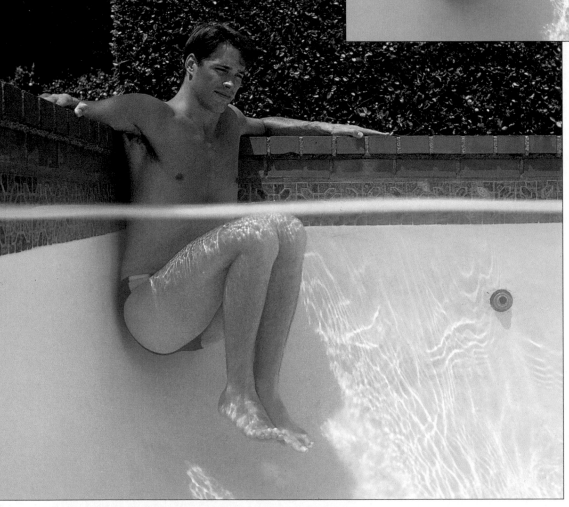

For an aquatic version of a sit-up, place your back against a corner of the pool, using your outstretched arms for support. Tuck your knees into your chest *(above)*, then forcefully push your legs straight out so that they are parallel to the pool bottom *(inset)*.

For this more difficult sit-up variation, support yourself with your outstretched arms, this time along a straight side of the pool. Tuck your legs into your chest *(below)*, then push them straight out from your hips *(bottom)*.

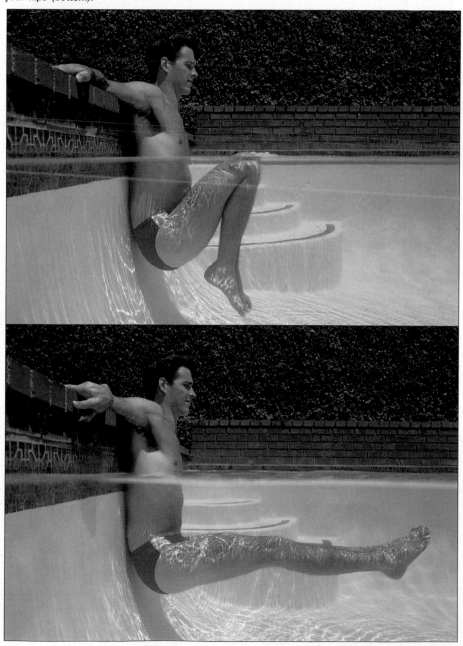

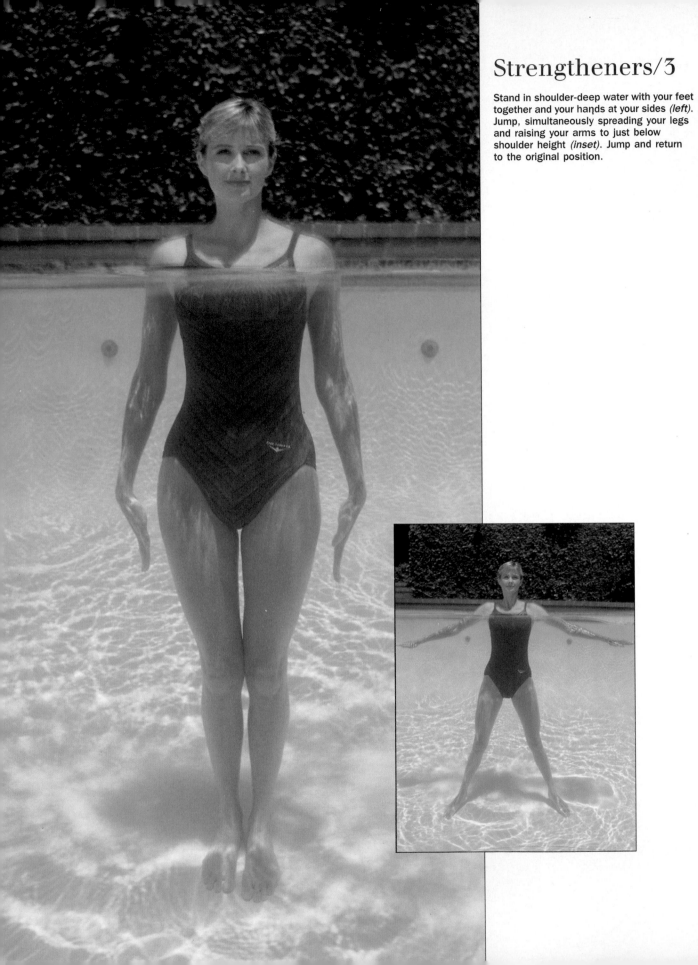

Strengtheners/3

Stand in shoulder-deep water with your feet together and your hands at your sides *(left)*. Jump, simultaneously spreading your legs and raising your arms to just below shoulder height *(inset)*. Jump and return to the original position.

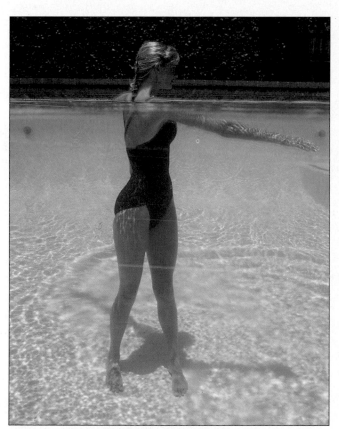
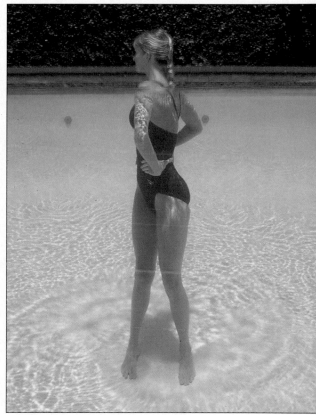

Stand in shoulder-deep water with your feet
slightly spread and your arms outstretched.
Swing your arms around as you twist your
torso first to the left *(above)*, then to the
right. Then put your hands on your hips and
twist both to your right and left *(right)*.

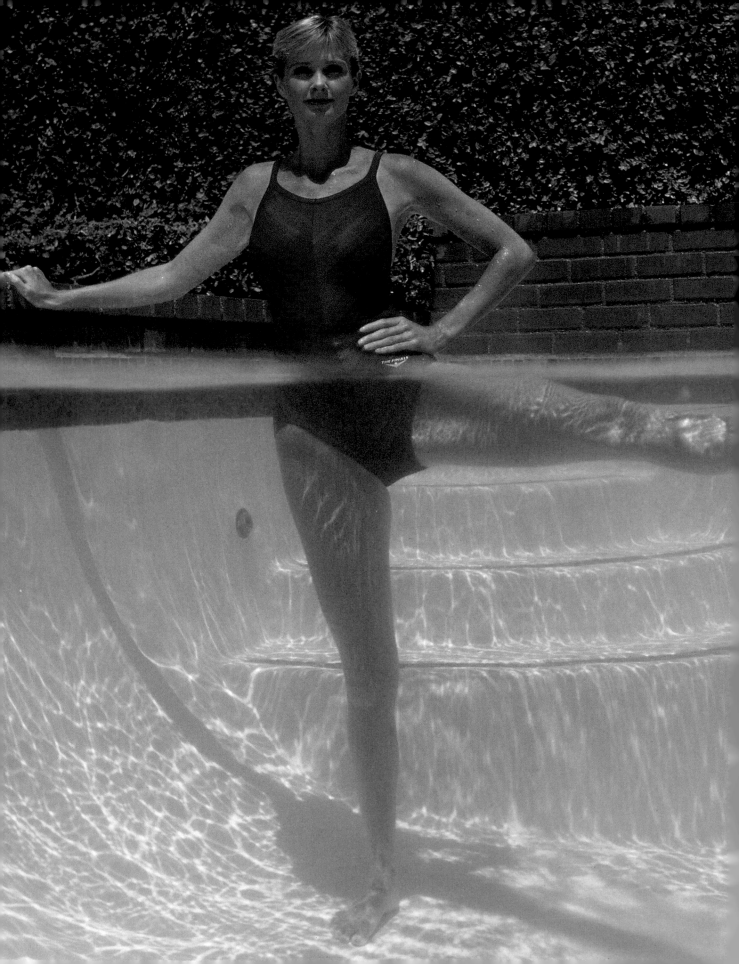

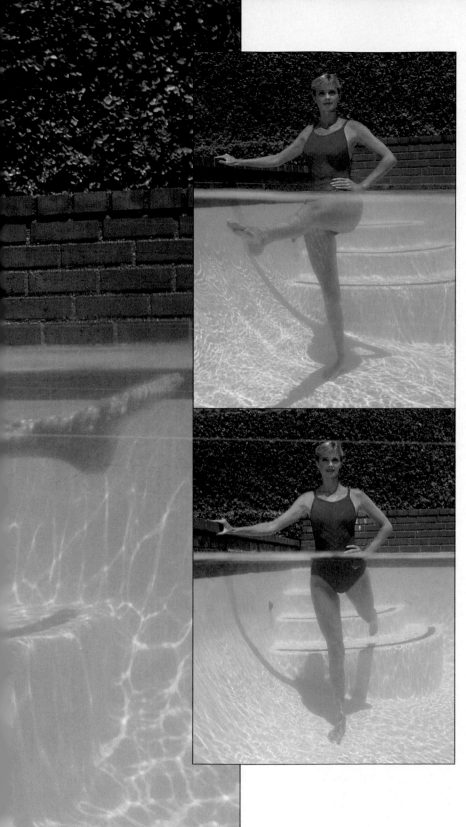

Stretches/1

Stand at arm's length from the edge of the pool in waist-high water. Grasp the edge with your right hand and place your left hand at your waist. Lift your left leg sideways to hip height *(opposite)*. Bring it forward, again at hip height *(left)*, then backward *(below)*. Reverse sides and repeat.

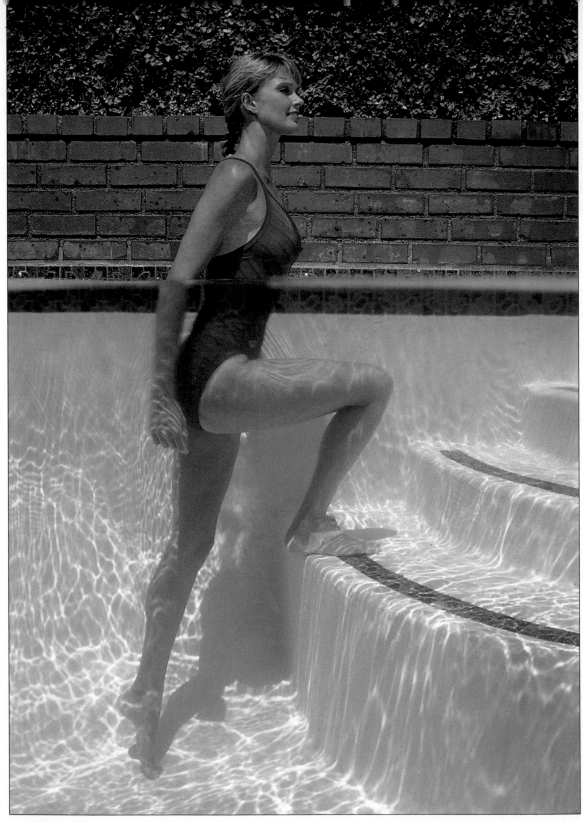

You will need a pool with steps for this exercise. Place your right foot on the bottom step and lean forward. Reverse legs.

Stretches/2

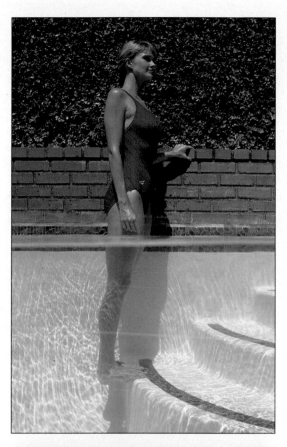

Stand with the balls of your feet on the bottom step of the pool stairs; hold on to the pool edge with your hand. Let your heels drop back; hold momentarily. Rise back up and repeat.

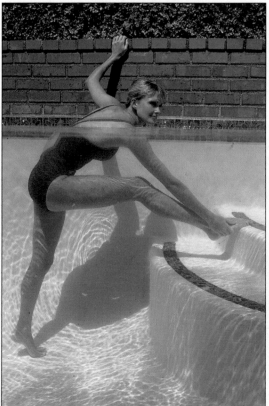

Grasp the edge of the pool and stand an arm's length away. Place your right foot on a step that is about thigh high. Extend your right leg and lean forward over it. Repeat with your left leg.

Aerobics/1

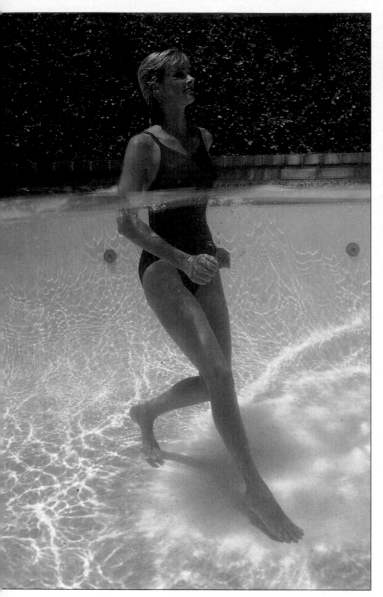

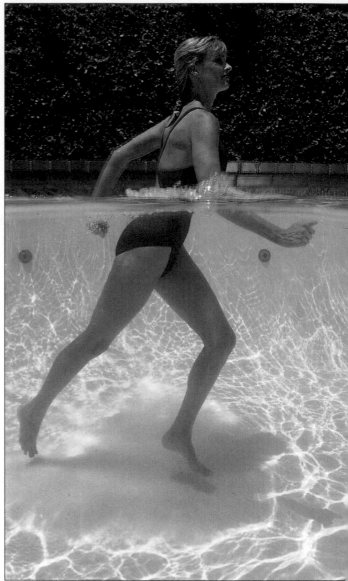

Stand in waist-deep water and run backward. Keep your back straight and pump your arms as you run.

Run forward in waist-deep water. Hold your chest high and pump your arms to maintain an upright position.

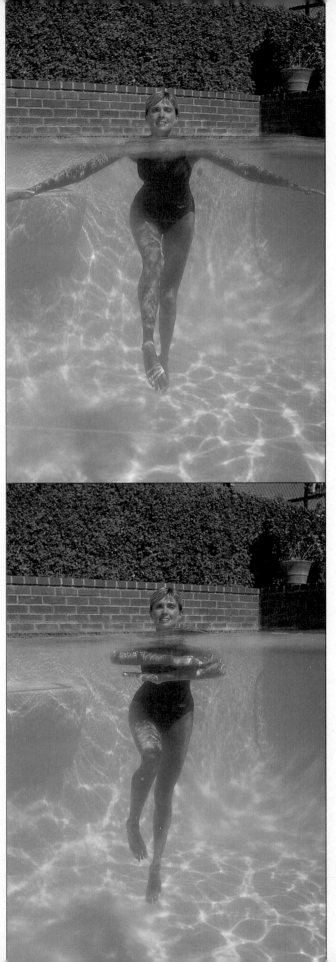

In addition to being a lifesaving skill, treading water is a good aerobic exercise that can be sustained for long periods. Perform this exercise in neck-deep water until you are comfortable and then tread water that is over your head. Pump your legs continuously as if you were on a bicycle; repeatedly extend your arms *(left)*, then bend your elbows to cross them in front of your chest *(below)*.

Aerobics/2

Stand in chest-deep water and link your
hands behind your head. Bend your left
knee and lift your leg to hip height as you
twist your torso, bringing your right elbow to
your knee *(right)*. Drop your left knee and
bring up your right, touching it to your left
elbow *(below)*.

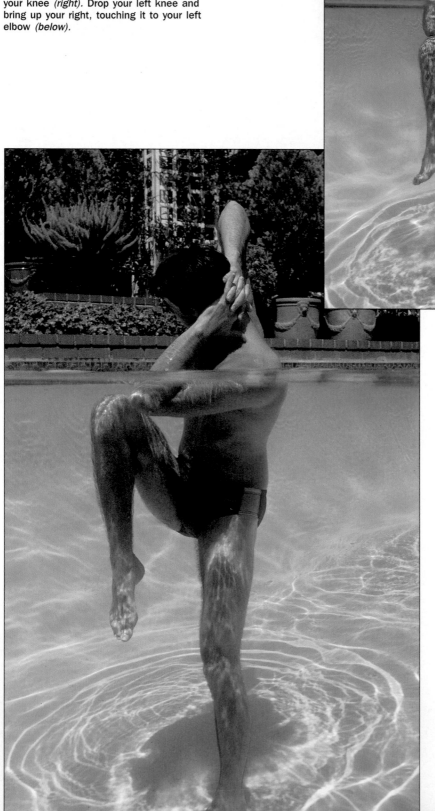

Stand in shoulder-deep water with your
elbows bent at your sides. Rotate your
wrists and jump up and down as if you
were twirling a jump rope.

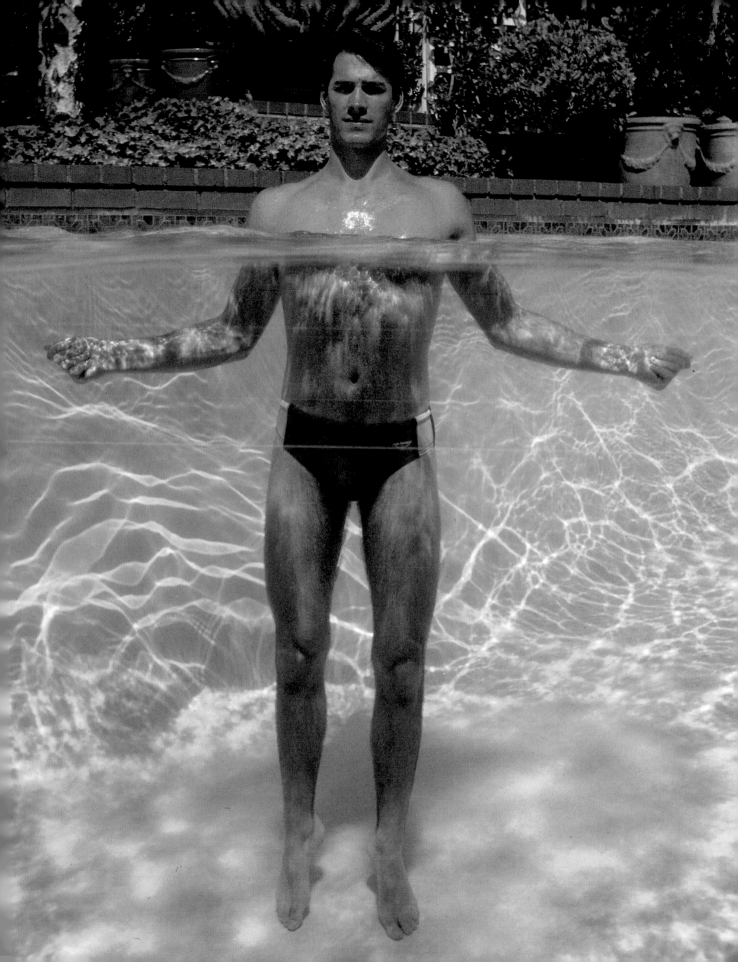

Swimming Maneuvers/1

A complete water workout should include swimming: Not only is it an effective cardiovascular conditioner and an excellent muscle toner, but it can also contribute the important elements of coordination and agility to your fitness program.

The exercises on these two pages and the following four isolate some of the arm and leg motions utilized in swimming. Concentrating individually on these specific maneuvers will help you to perfect them, as well as condition the muscles used in swimming. Perform each of the strokes and kicks for at least one minute. Then combine them and add 15 minutes or more of lap work to your water workout.

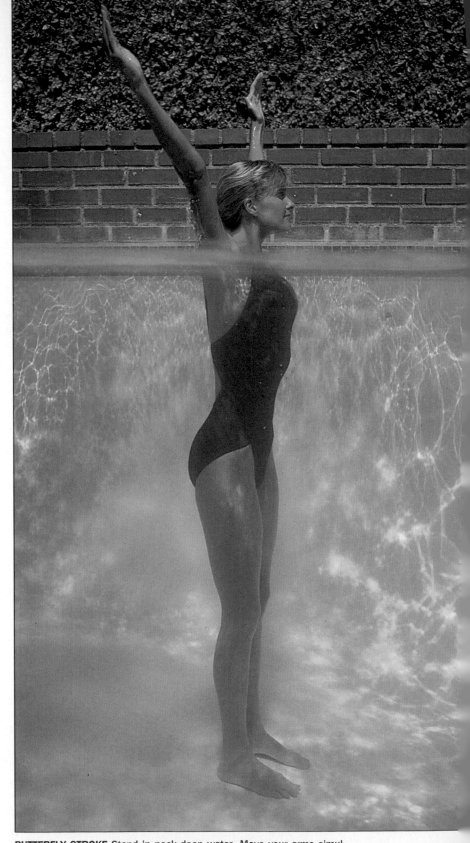

BUTTERFLY STROKE Stand in neck-deep water. Move your arms simultaneously, each arm curving outward, then inward to your sides as they enter the water. Follow by using alternate arms to make an S-shape pull, which is the freestyle stroke.

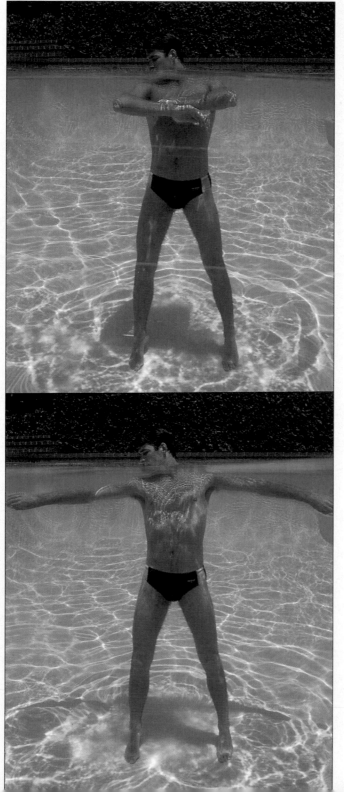

SIDESTROKE Stand in neck-deep water. Move your arms in opposite motions, one arm pulling and one pushing. Turn your head so that it tilts to the right side and tuck your arms in front of your chest with your hands cupped outward *(left).* Push backward with your left arm, letting your right arm glide forward *(bottom).* Then pull toward your chest with your right arm as your left arm glides back. Tilt your head to the left and repeat for your left side.

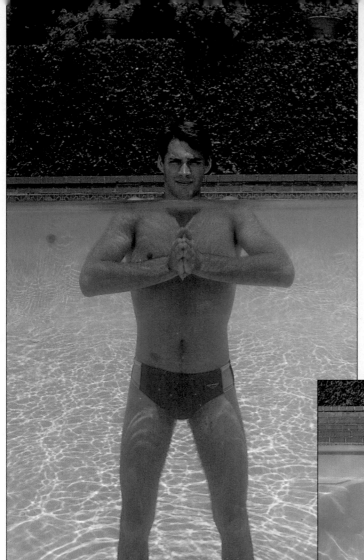

Swimming Maneuvers/2

BREASTSTROKE Bend your arms so that your hands touch and point outward in front of your chest *(left)*. Move your hands forward, then gradually separate your arms, cupping your hands to push the water away from you *(below)*. Extend your arms all the way out to your sides *(bottom)*, then bend your elbows and bring them back into your chest in a heart-shaped motion.

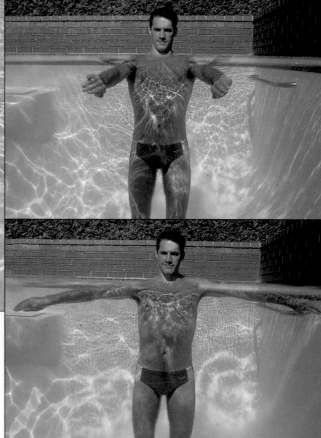

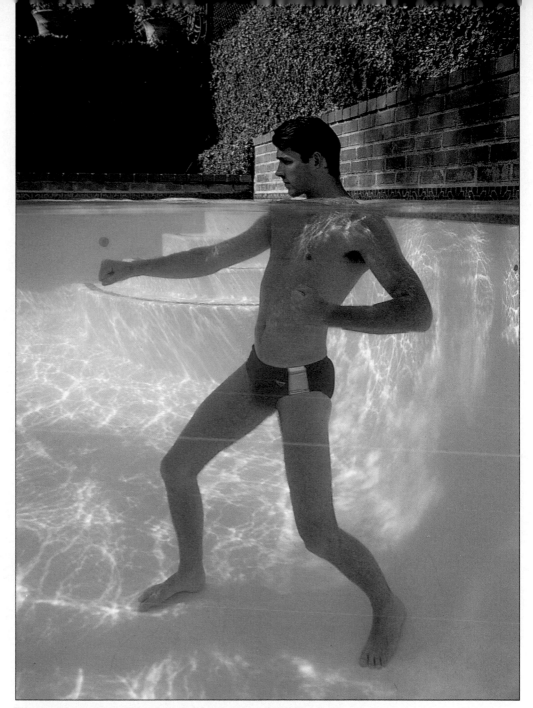

This exercise uses water resistance to build up the arm strength necessary
for effective swimming strokes. Spread your legs and forcefully punch
the water in front of you with alternating arms.

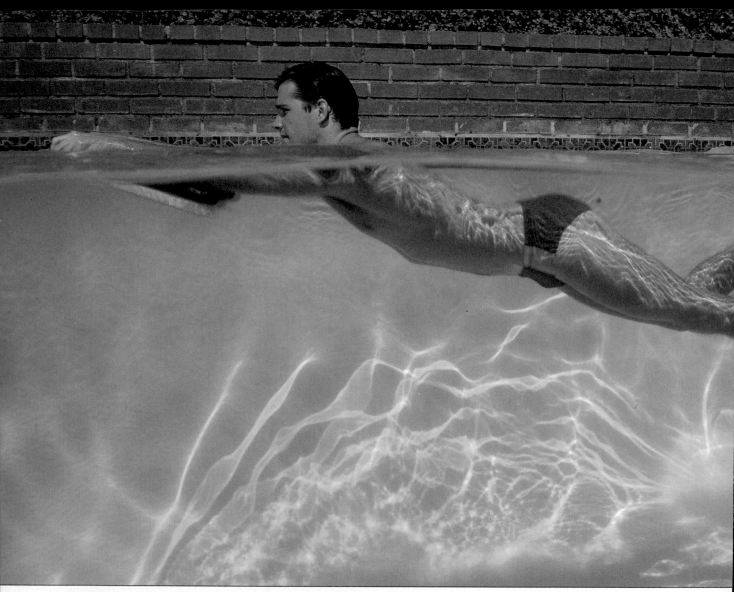

FLUTTER KICK You can either use a kickboard or hold on to the edge of the pool to practice kicking movements. Stretch your legs out straight behind you with your ankles relaxed and your toes pointed. Alternately kick your legs, letting the motion come from your hip *(above)*.

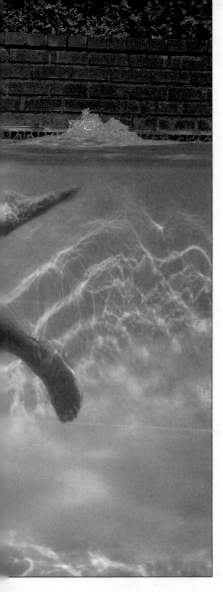

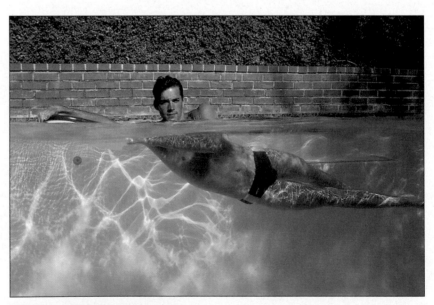

SCISSORS KICK Begin with your legs
together and your toes pointed. Bring your
knees toward your chest, then back down as
you separate and straighten your legs in a
wide V shape *(above)*. Then bring your
legs back together.

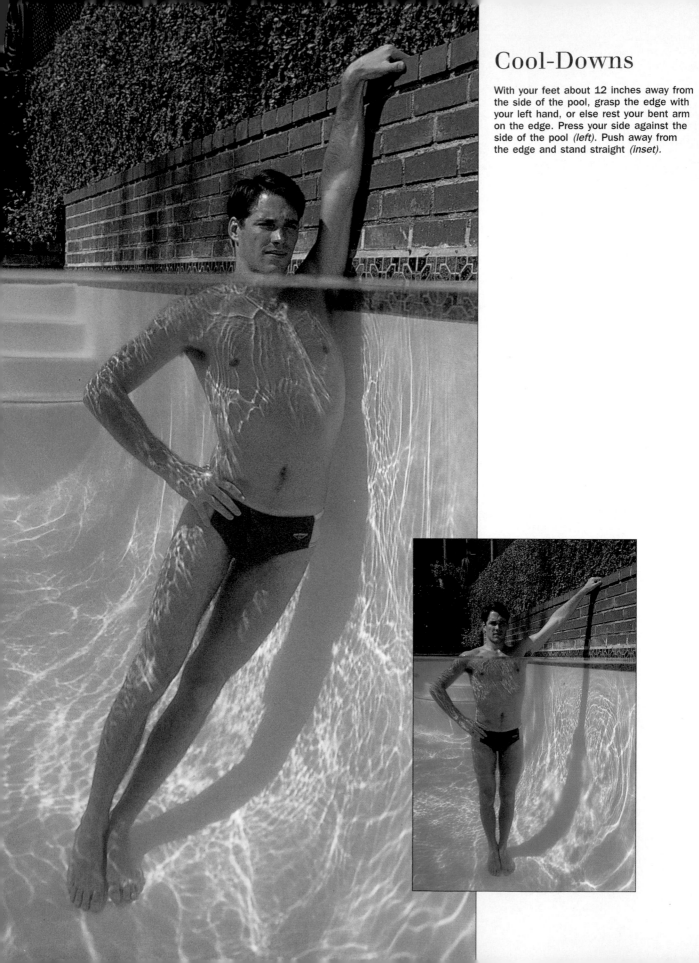

Cool-Downs

With your feet about 12 inches away from the side of the pool, grasp the edge with your left hand, or else rest your bent arm on the edge. Press your side against the side of the pool *(left)*. Push away from the edge and stand straight *(inset)*.

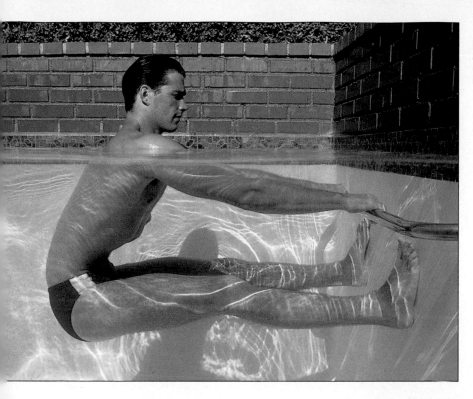

If your pool has a bar, grip it; otherwise, grasp the gutter. Bring your feet up against the pool just beneath your hands and extend your arms and legs. Hold.

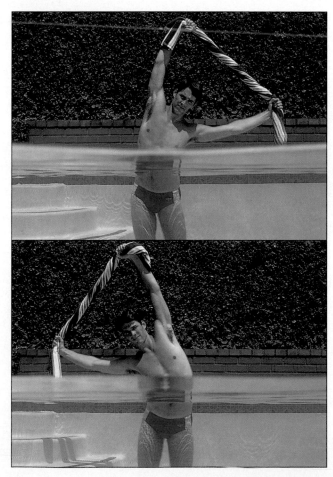

Hold a rolled towel at either end and bend to your left *(top)*, then to your right *(right)*.

97

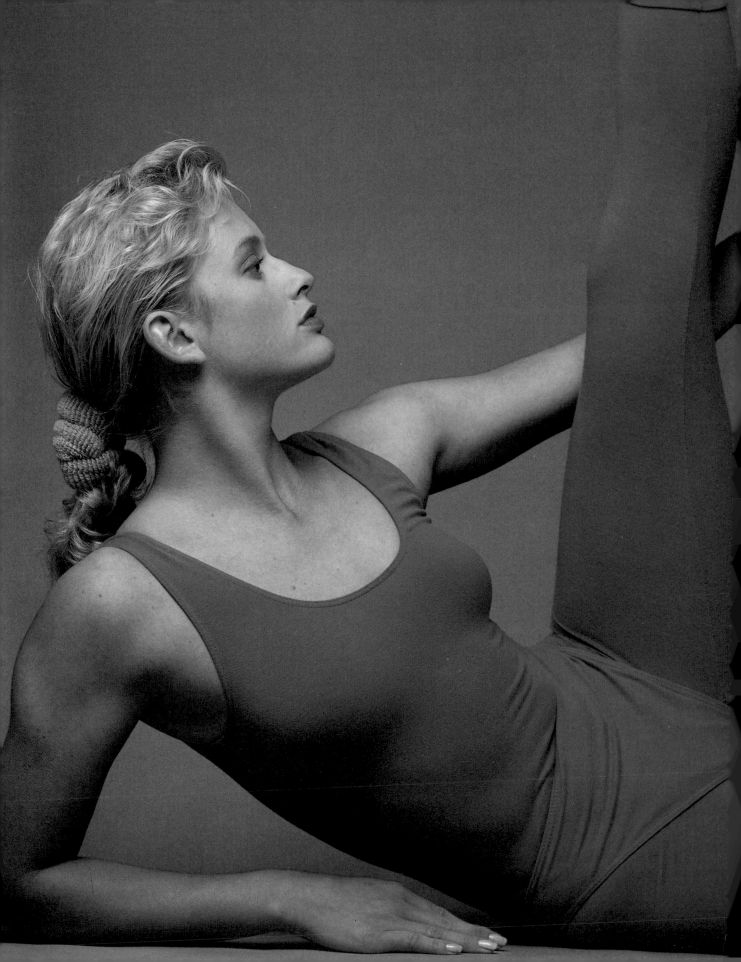

CHAPTER FOUR

Movement

Low-impact routines for developing your natural grace and agility

O ne of the best ways of softening the impact of any exercise is to take advantage of the body's natural movement patterns. Understanding what happens to your body when you undertake physical activity is the basis for movement theory, whose proponents have developed special motion sequences to improve coordination, flexibility and agility.

The scientific underpinning of movement theory is kinesiology, which draws on the physical sciences — particularly physics, anatomy and physiology — to examine the ways in which human bodies move. By applying to the body the mechanical principles of balance, equilibrium and the application of force, kinesiologists try to explain the operational requirements of motion.

Kinesiologists view the body as a machine whose movements are coordinated and can be mapped. For example, a kinesiologist will determine how the laws of motion apply to the activity of running in order to understand the mechanics of acceleration and forward propulsion. Comprehending which mechanisms control the body's operation and how they do it can be a means to revising ineffective movement patterns. This approach allows the kinesiologist to create an ideal model for running that can be used to improve an individual runner's technique.

Like kinesiologists, movement therapists seek to understand how individual muscles and parts of the body function within the context of the whole system. However, they do not study the body through the biomechanical lens of the kinesiologist. While both kinesiologists and movement therapists base their suggestions for improvements on their analysis of a subject, movement therapists view this process as educational as well as diagnostic. Thus, they encourage the individual to examine his or her own patterns of moving from another perspective — an internal one. Such an analysis requires that the individual develop an awareness of not only his or her bodily sensations, but also how he or she uses the surrounding space.

Much of the graceful motion associated with childhood is lost as you age, when you may find yourself forced into prolonged periods of sitting or standing. To counteract this, movement therapists use routines that recreate the development of gross motor skills in the human body. By imitating the progression of human physical development from lying down to rolling over, standing, pivoting and walking, movement sequences can help improve performance of basic activities.

Any time the body moves, there is a primary and usually intentional action coupled with secondary, or complementary actions, usually meant to balance the body. The primary muscular action of throwing a ball, for example, occurs in the throwing arm. Secondary actions in the legs and torso maintain the body's balance. Movement therapists treat every bodily function as part of a comprehensive effort. For example, although a sit-up is primarily an exercise for the abdominals, it requires the coordinated effort of your back, head, arms and legs. Movement therapists claim that such exercise performed without an understanding of the interactions of the entire body can be ineffectual and sometimes dangerous. Thus, they do not prescribe exercises for single body parts. Rather, they create sequences that require concentration on the secondary action as well as on the primary action. Performing sequences such as the walk-around on pages 120-121, which emphasizes the proper alignment between the head and the pelvis, and the roundabout on pages 114-115, which necessitates complementary use of leg and abdominal muscles, will develop your awareness of the careful body coordination required for even a relatively simple motion.

In the movement sequences on the following eight pages, the entire routines are performed in a standing, sitting or kneeling position. When you become proficient at these, you can progress to the more advanced sequences, starting on page 110, that incorporate the element of transition — shifting from sitting to standing and sometimes back to the floor — and so require working with gravity.

Movement Fundamentals

> Maintain a slight contraction of your abdominal muscles. These muscles provide support for both your upper and lower body and help forces generated in the lower body to be transferred to the upper body and vice versa; for example, the arm movement for throwing a ball is initiated by taking a step, and contracted abdominals will aid in this transfer of force. Contracted abdominals also help protect your lower back from overuse and strain. The roundabout *(pages 114-115)* is strongly dependent on this principle for its successful execution.

> Coordinate your breathing with exertion. As part of the mechanism of breathing, exhaling facilitates the contraction of your abdominals. The spider *(pages 110-111)* is a good exercise to practice this technique with.

> Strive for full rotation of the hip and shoulder joints. These ball-and-socket joints are designed to move in a full circular range, and mobility in the hip and shoulder can prevent lower back or neck strain. Ineffective movement patterns frequently substitute use of the lower back, knees and neck for movement that ought to occur in the hip or shoulder. To facilitate full range of motion in the shoulder, turn your palm upward when you move your arm in front of your body; when you move your arm behind you, turn the palm downward. Practice these arm rotations in the serve *(pages 106-107)* and the cantilever *(pages 122-123)*. To enhance rotation of the hip, turn the inside of your thigh upward when moving your leg forward, and downward toward the floor when moving your leg behind you. Both leg-threading *(pages 102-103)* and the crawl-around *(pages 108-109)* rely on full hip rotation.

> Move your upper and lower body in opposing directions to maintain balance. This important principle, called counterbalance, establishes equilibrium in motion. Balance is not static; for example, as your arm moves forward, one of your legs will move back. Counterbalance can be maintained in many different configurations: up and down, the basic balancing movement you use when getting up from a chair and which is used in the walk-around *(pages 120-121)*; forward and backward, seen in the cantilever *(pages 122-123)*; side to side, a movement in the figure 8 *(pages 116-117)*; and diagonal counterbalance, demonstrated in the crossover *(pages 112-113)*.

> Keep your elbows and knees unlocked. This allows movement to flow from your extremities to the torso, and vice versa.

Routines such as side circling on pages 118-119 require careful balance and coordination to complete the transitions successfully.

The movement skills you will acquire from these sequences can be used to improve other activities or exercises. For example, the pitch and the serve sequences on pages 106-107 are designed to duplicate use of the muscles in baseball, softball and racquet sports. In addition, all of the sequences encourage full joint mobility, which in turn allows muscles to work more efficiently. This can dramatically reduce the effort — and possible injury — inherent in many forms of exercise. Many athletic strains and injuries result from overuse of the neck, lower back and knees because of a lack of shoulder and hip-joint mobility. The sequences in this chapter encourage the full use of these joints, thus distributing the stress on the body more evenly.

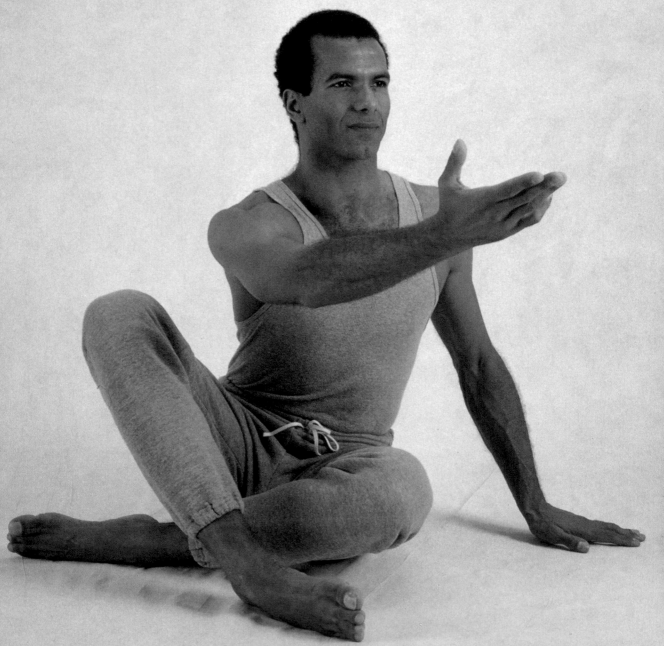

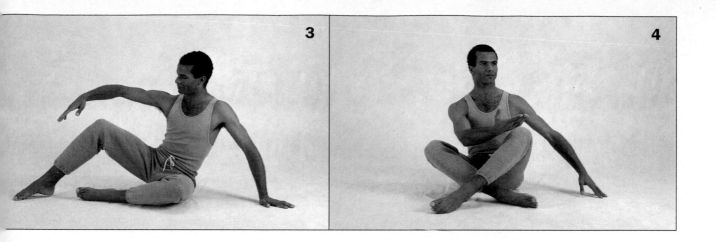

The Basic Routines

The goal of movement routines is not to build strength or endurance through increased repetitions or longer workout sessions, as many exercise programs aim to do. Instead, the object is to develop an understanding of the interactions among parts of the body. For example, many of the following routines emphasize coordination of the head with the pelvis. These separate body parts must function interdependently to help ensure proper posture.

Mastering such techniques can help improve your performance in other physical endeavors. Initiating leg movement with hip-joint rotation, as the routine on these two pages does, can give you insight into the biomechanical requirements for activities like kicking a soccer ball or

doing the breaststroke — both of which use the hip joint.

In order to benefit from these routines, you should practice them slowly and precisely; only in that way can you become aware of the coordination of your body in movement.

The following five sequences are relatively simple because each is confined to one basic posture: sitting, standing, kneeling or lying. Work on a mat or a thick carpet.

You should aim for smooth, flowing motion from step to step. Performing the routines in front of a mirror might help you to evaluate your movements.

Perform each routine two or three times. And with sequences that are shown for only one side of the body, be sure to repeat them on the other side as well.

LEG THREADING Sit cross-legged on the floor. Support yourself with your left arm as you raise your right knee and extend your right arm in front of you (1). Rotate your right arm and right leg to the right side (2). Curve your outstretched arm downward, as you bend your right knee up (3). Thread your right foot under your left leg and return your right arm to its original position (4).

Windmill

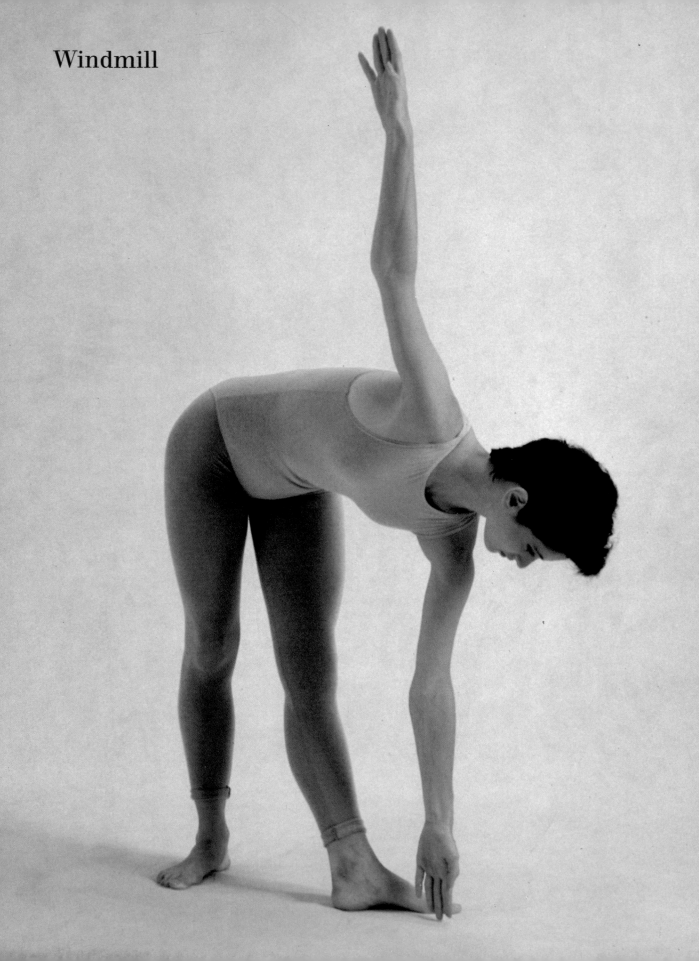

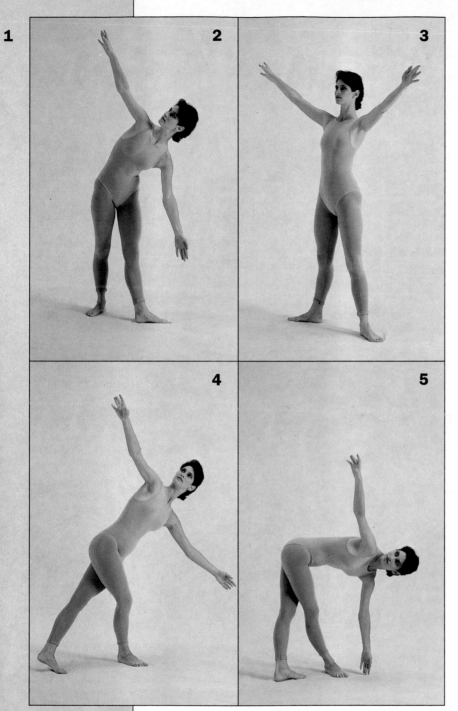

Stand with your feet spread slightly and at right angles to each other, your left foot in front. Lean forward to touch the floor in front of your left foot with the fingertips of your left hand, keeping both arms fully extended, with your right arm behind you (1). Slowly unbend and reach your right arm upward (2), rising to an erect posture with arms outstretched and feet spread (3). Pivot 180 degrees on your right foot, bringing your left foot behind you (4), then bend over to touch the floor with your left hand. Your right arm should extend upward again (5).

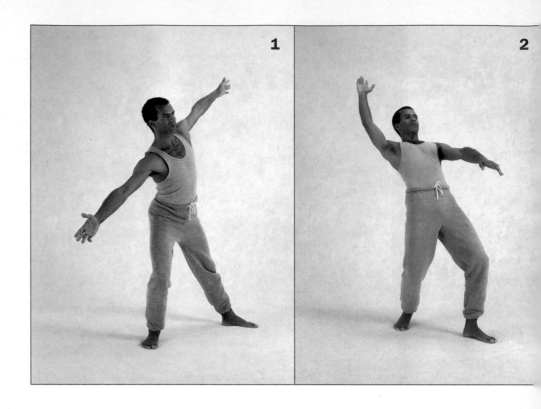

Pitch

Stand up straight, then lean onto your
right leg, letting your left **foot** lift slightly,
and reach up with your right arm (1).
Bring your left foot forward and lean back
on your right leg, dropping your arm (2).
Then shift your weight onto your left leg as
you curve your right arm forward and raise
your right leg behind you (3).

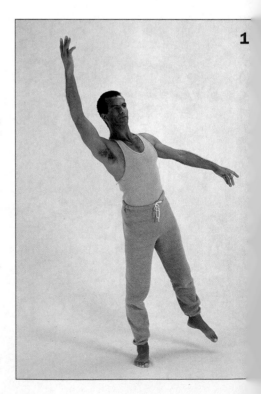

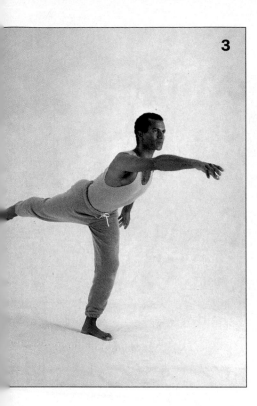

Serve

Stand with your feet spread wide and your arms outstretched. Bend your right knee slightly and lean to the right (1). Lean backward, moving your right leg and right arm back, and extend your left arm in front of you (2). Thrust your right arm forward smoothly, lifting your right leg as you shift your weight onto your left (3).

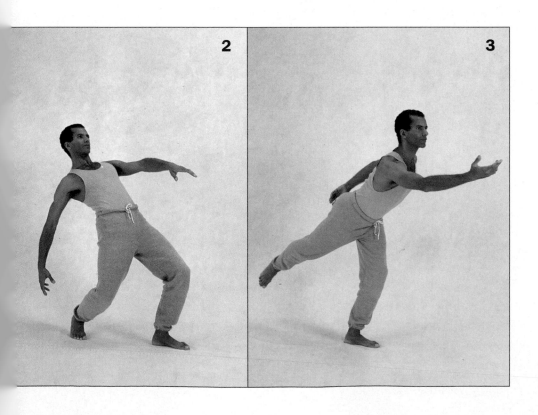

Crawl-Around

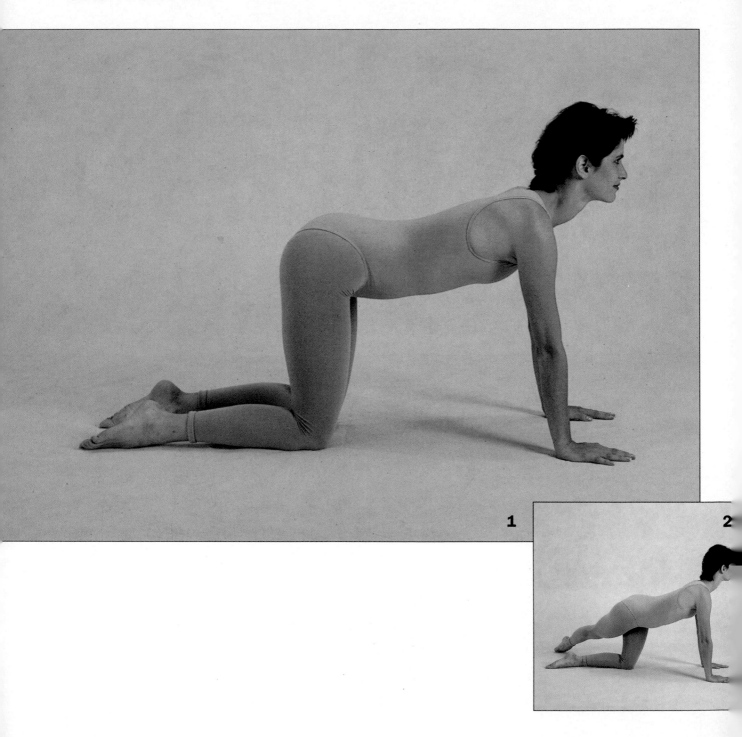

1

2

Kneel on all fours, keeping your back flat
(1). Extend your right leg, crossing it over
your left (2). Swing the right leg out to
your right side so that it forms a right
angle when you bend your knee (3). Cross
your right leg in front of your left and drop
the knee to the floor (4). Raise your left
leg and bring it over the right and return
to the starting position (5).

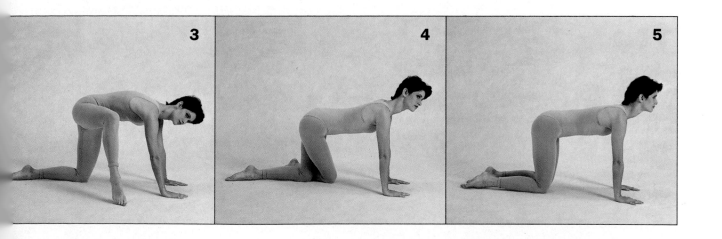

Adding Transitions

Once you have mastered the sequences on pages 102-109, you are ready to move on to more advanced routines. These incorporate transitions that call for you to shift postures from standing to sitting to lying. The shifts require you to compensate for the pull of gravity — for example, pro-pulsion is necessary to push off on one leg and stand up from a kneeling position, and momentum is needed to roll up from a lying to a sitting posture.

Do not try to perform all these routines immediately. Concentrate on perfecting two or three exercises before working on a new one.

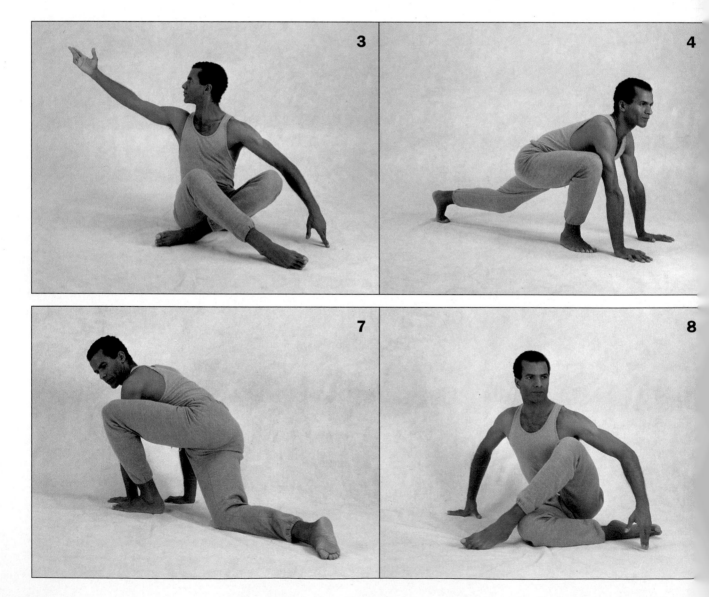

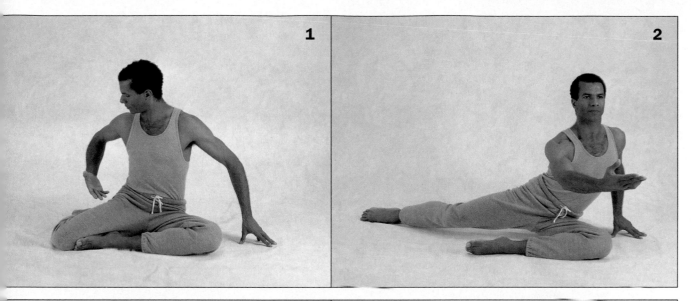

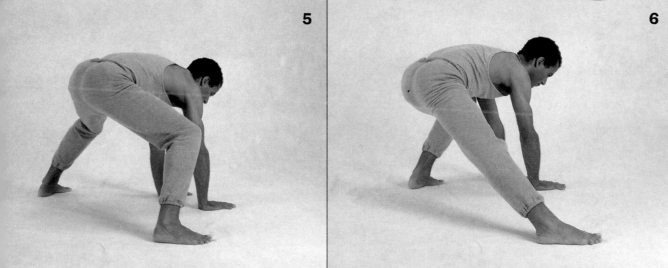

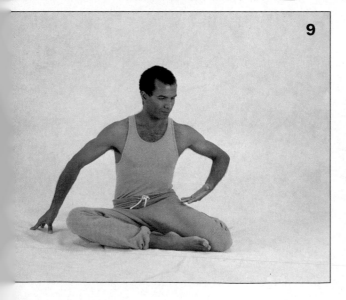

SPIDER Sit with your left leg bent in front of you and your right leg bent back at the knee. Support yourself on your left arm and curve your right arm (1). Bring your right arm forward as you extend your right leg back (2). Cross your right leg in front of you and reach your right arm behind you (3), then, supporting yourself on your hands in front of you, shift your weight forward onto your bent right leg and extend your left leg behind you (4). Shift your weight from your right to your left leg through a squatting position (5), extending your right leg sideways (6). Pivot your hips to fold your right knee underneath you (7). Continue turning to lower yourself to a seated position with your left leg bent across your right (8). Circle your left leg to the side and bend it behind you (9).

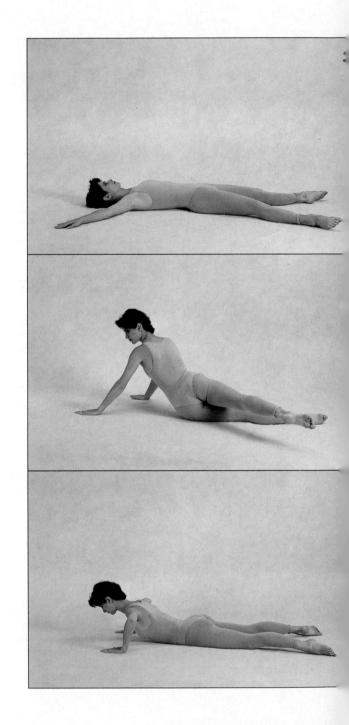

Crossover

Lie flat on your back with your arms and legs outstretched (1). Reach your right arm across your body to roll onto your right side (2), then to a prone position (3). Reach your right leg behind you to roll to your left, simultaneously pushing up with your arms (4), then twist to a sitting position with your right leg extended and your left leg folded in front of you (5). Turn your torso over your right leg, and extend your arms in front of you (6). Keep twisting your torso to the right, extending your legs behind you and supporting yourself on your arms as you roll again to a prone position (7). Extend your arms to push your torso up and turn to your left (8), rising to sit with your right leg folded in front and your left leg and your right arm extended.

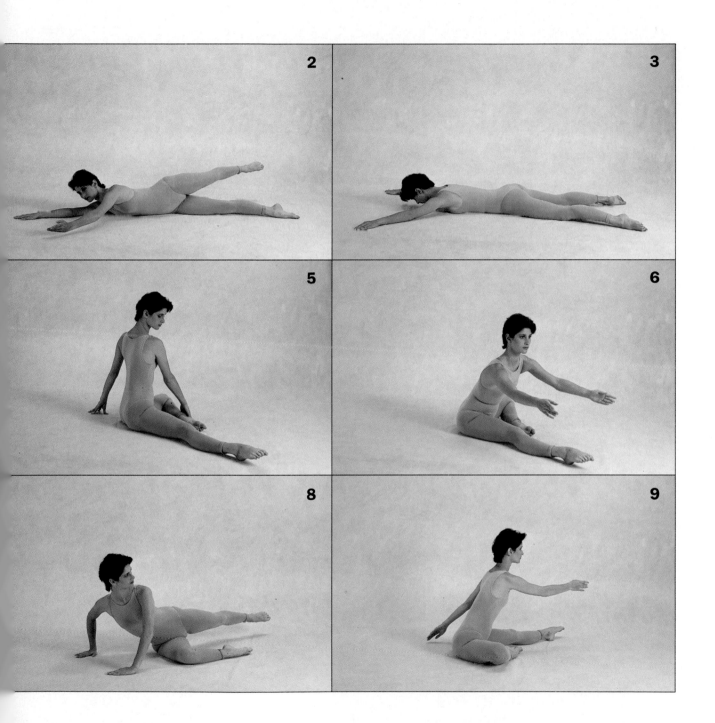

Roundabout

Lean on your arms with your legs outstretched to your left (1).
Lift your left arm and pivot onto your hip (2) to swing your legs
directly in front of you, keeping your feet slightly raised off the
floor (3). Continue pivoting and moving your legs, shifting your
weight to your left arm (4), then twisting your body forward
onto both arms (5), as your legs rotate behind you (6).
Straighten your arms as you cross your right leg, knee bent,
behind you (7). Continue turning your torso until you sit facing
the opposite direction from where you began (8).

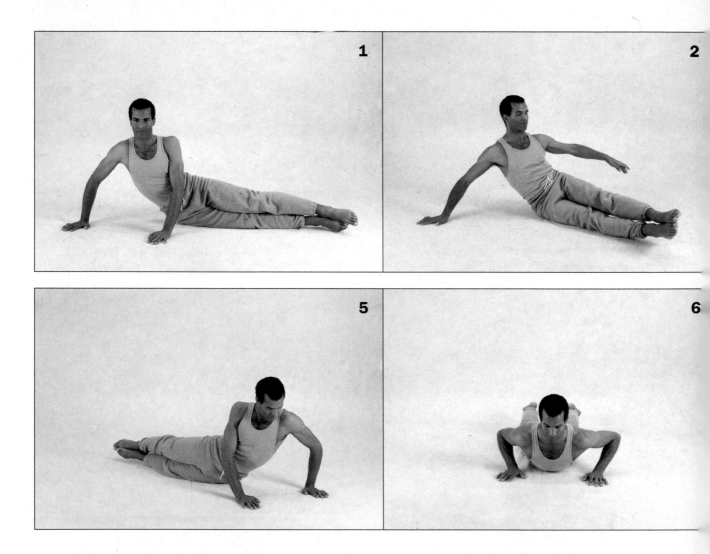

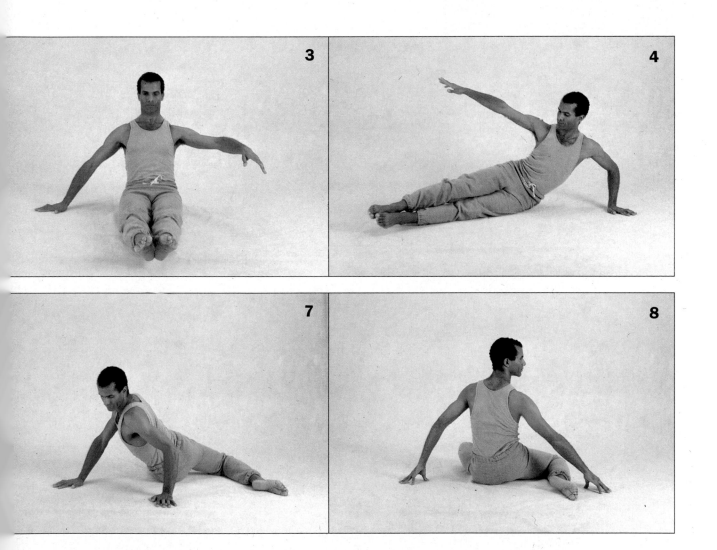

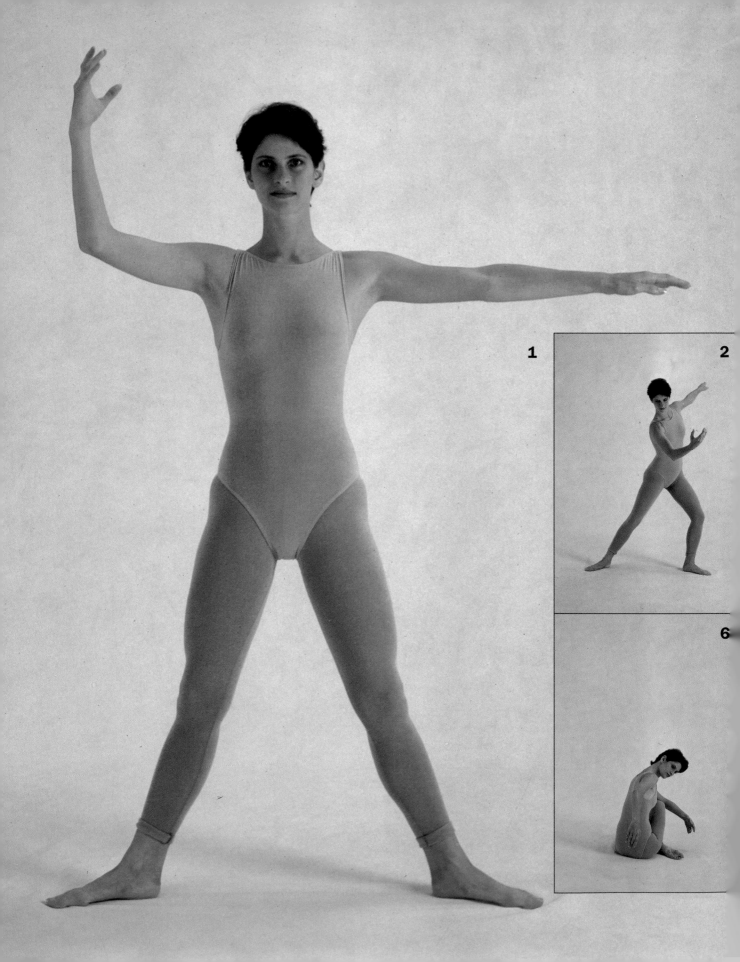

Figure 8

Stand with your feet spread apart, your left arm extended and your right arm bent at the elbow (1). Shift your weight to the left, crossing your right arm in front of you (2), then bend both knees (3) and swing both your arms to the right, allowing your torso to shift over your right leg (4). Keep rotating your arms to the right as you bend your left knee (5) and fold yourself into a cross-legged sit (6). Next, swing your arms to the left and unfold your legs (7), pivoting on your right leg (8). Center your weight as you rise to your original position (9).

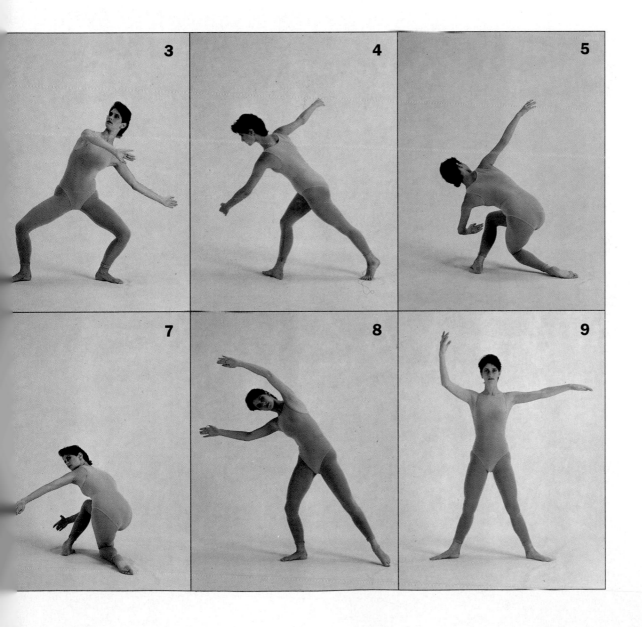

Side Circling

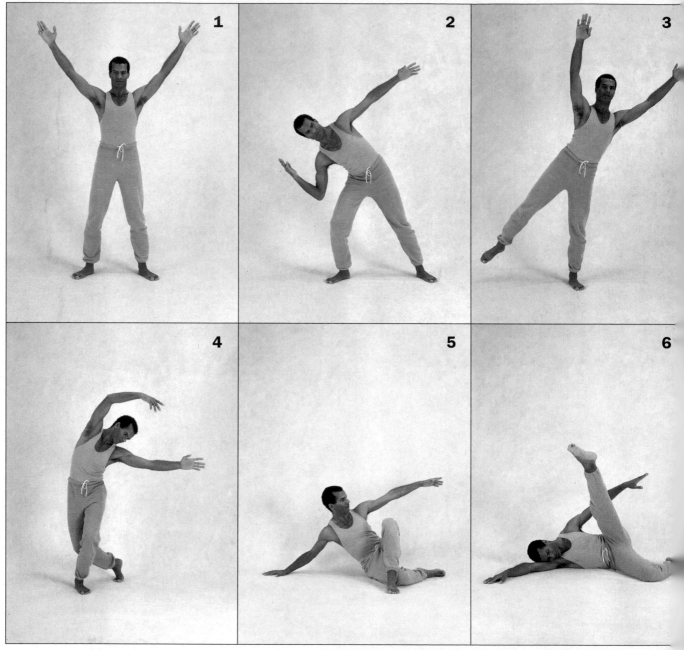

Stand with your legs apart and your arms outstretched (1). Bend your right elbow and bring it down to your bent right knee (2). Extend both arms as you push off with your right foot, shift your weight and lean to the left (3). Bring your bent right leg behind your left leg (4). Lean back to your right and slide down onto your right side (5). Stretch out on your right side as you raise your left leg (6), then lower it and use the momentum to rise onto your right knee (7). Continue to propel yourself forward to a stand (8).

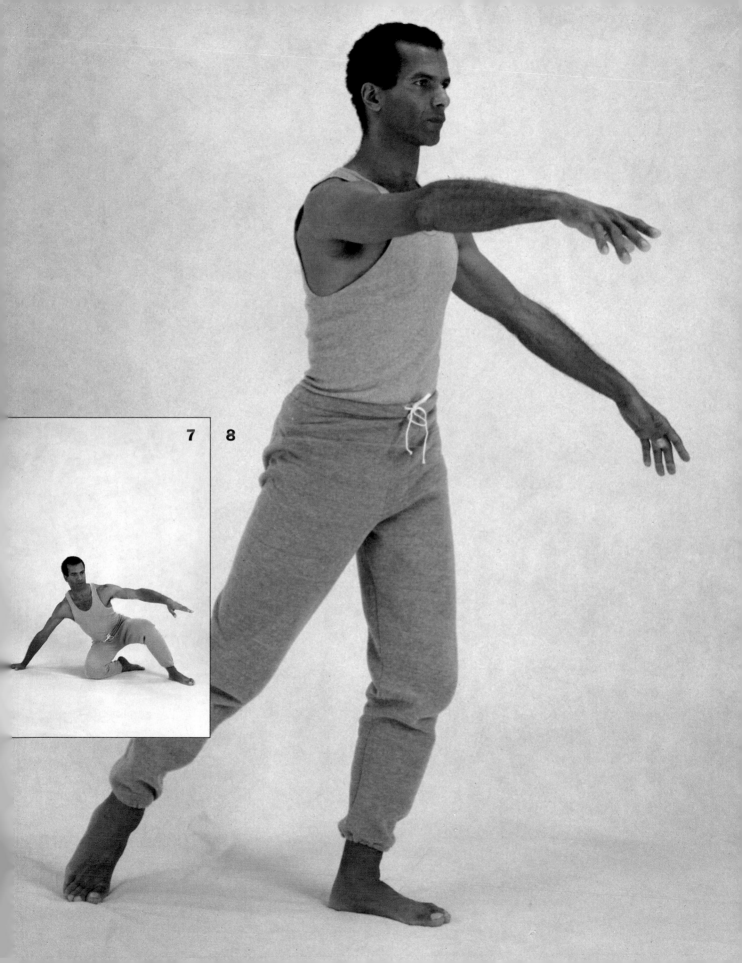

7   8

Walk-Around

Stand with your feet apart and raise your arms above your head (1). Lower your arms and drop into a crouch position (2), then thrust your body forward, supporting yourself on your outstretched arms (3). Twist at your waist so your feet are in contact with the floor and take small steps forward (4), bringing your right arm behind you and your legs in front of you into a "table" position (5). Bend at the hip joint and take small steps backward to "walk" your legs underneath you, returning to a crouch position (6). Keep your hands on the floor as you straighten your legs as far as you can (7).

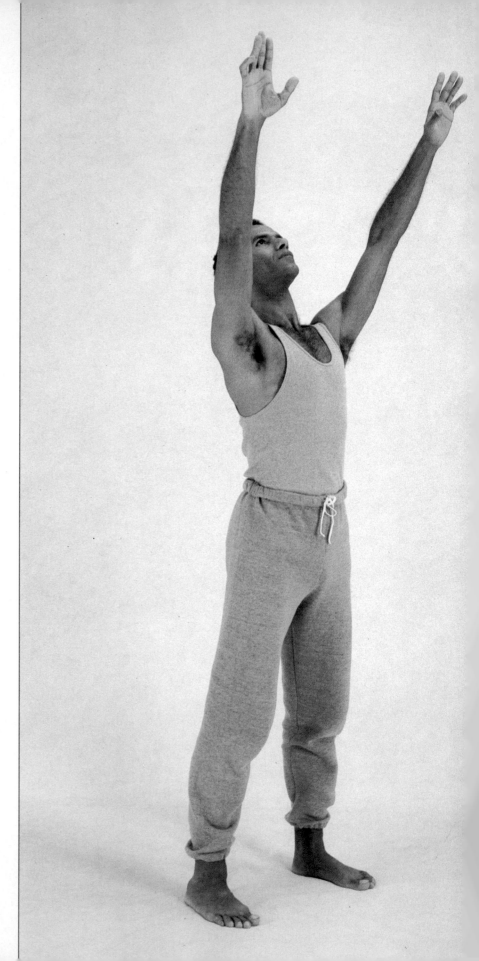

1

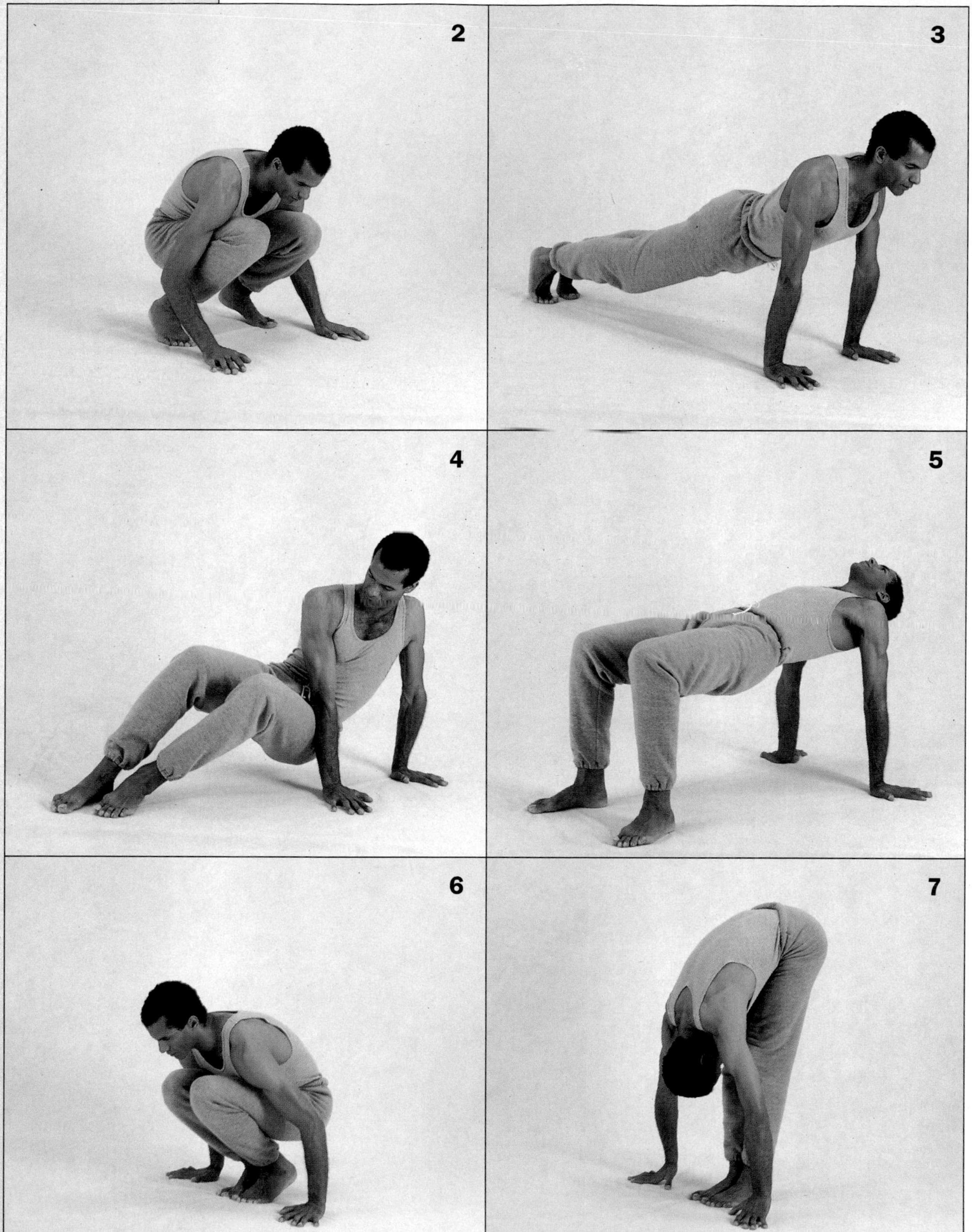

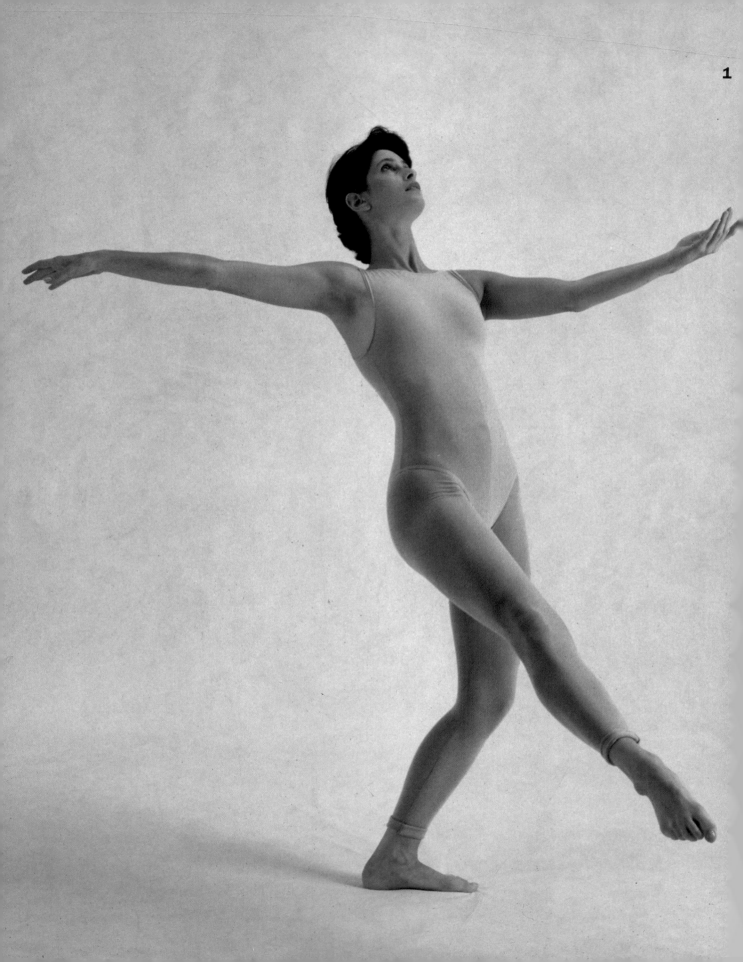

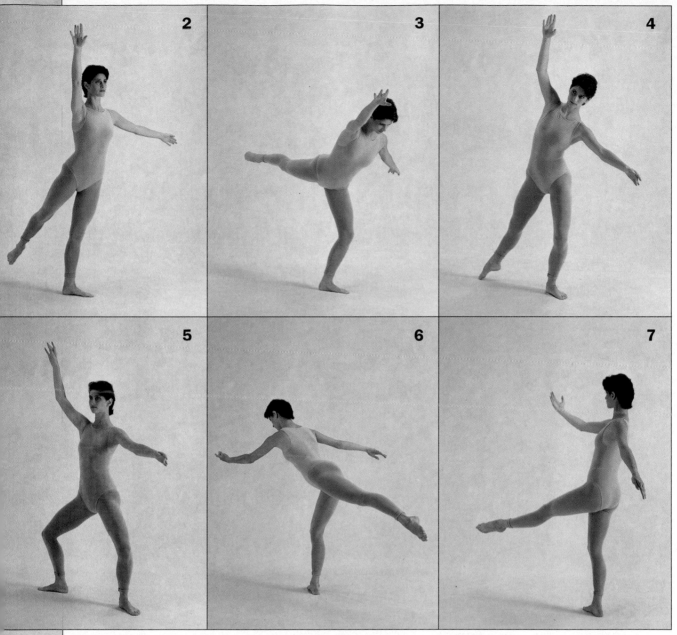

Cantilever

Lean slightly backward with your left knee bent, your right foot raised in front of you and your arms outstretched (1). Shift your weight and lean forward as you swing your right leg back (2) and right arm forward (3). Raise your torso and turn to the right, touching your right foot to the floor (4), then distribute your weight evenly between your legs in a plié position (5). Shift weight onto your right leg, bringing your left leg back and left arm forward (6). Swing your left leg and right arm forward (7).

RECOMMENDED DAILY ALLOWANCES

Vitamin A is given in retinol equivalents (RE), which measure the vitamin A that you actually absorb, whether you consume retinol (the usable form of vitamin A from animal sources) or beta carotene (the vitamin A precursor from plant foods that your body converts to retinol). One RE is equal to one milligram of retinol or six milligrams of beta carotene. The Recommended Daily Allowance (RDA) is 800 RE for women and 1,000 for men — amounts supplied by one large carrot.

Vitamin D is measured in micrograms. The RDA for both men and women is 10 micrograms, which can be supplied by one ounce of sardines.

Vitamin E, which exists in several slightly different chemical forms, is measured in tocopherol equivalents (TE); tocopherol is another name for the vitamin. One milligram of vitamin E equals one TE. The RDA is 10 TE for men and eight for women, both of which are supplied by 1/2 ounce of corn oil.

No RDA has been determined for vitamin K. The suggested intake is 70 to 140 micrograms per day, the amount contained in 1/4 cup of spinach.

vitamin also aids in the division and growth of body cells, helps maintain normal vision in dim light and protects the skin and the lining of the nose and throat from infection. In addition, some research indicates that people whose diets include plenty of vegetarian foods that supply vitamin A have a lower incidence of certain forms of cancer than people who consume less of these foods.

The vegetables that provide you with vitamin A do so through chemicals called carotenoids — vitamin A precursors that your body converts to vitamin A. The most abundant carotenoid is beta carotene, found in such vegetables and fruits as spinach, broccoli, sweet potatoes, carrots, squash, tomatoes, apricots and peaches. Vitamin A itself is found in generous amounts in egg yolks, dairy products, oily fish and liver — and it occurs not as a precursor, but in a form called retinol that your body uses directly. This does not mean, however, that these animal-derived foods are the best sources of vitamin A. A vegetarian dish like the Rosy Ratatouille on page 131 and a meat recipe such as the Chopped Liver Spread on page 139 both provide the recommended daily amount.

Animal-derived vitamin A is used in vitamin supplements, but anyone taking supplements should be careful. Doses that exceed 10 times the daily recommended allowance can be toxic, potentially causing tenderness or pain in bones as well as liver and brain damage. Beta carotene and other carotenoids, however, are not known to be toxic when you consume more than you need.

Vitamin D can be obtained from your diet, but it is also formed in your skin when you are exposed to sunlight. The regulation of calcium and phosphorus metabolism is vitamin D's most important role. It promotes the intestinal absorption of calcium, regulates the movement of calcium and phosphorus in and out of bones and teeth, and maintains the proper levels of these two minerals in the blood. By promoting an adequate blood level of calcium, vitamin D also ensures the proper functioning of the nerves and muscles.

Vitamin D occurs naturally in only a few common foodstuffs such as oily fish, liver, eggs and butter. However, milk and breakfast cereals are often fortified with this vitamin, and it is easy to work into recipes: The Carrot-Rice Pudding on page 138 and the Scandinavian-Style Canapés on page 140 contain ample amounts of vitamin D. No one should take vitamin D supplements without medical supervision, since doses that contain more than 10 times the daily recommended allowance are extremely toxic.

In contrast to vitamins A and D, vitamin E's functions are not well delineated, although many health and cosmetic claims have been made for it. What is known is that vitamin E acts as an antioxidant, a substance that keeps oxygen from combining with and altering fats. When fats contained in cell membranes react with oxygen, they break down into chemicals called peroxides, and, consequently, the cell membranes are destroyed.

Because of its antioxidant function, some researchers believe that

The Basic Guidelines

For a moderately active adult, the National Institutes of Health recommends a diet that is low in fat, high in carbohydrates and moderate in protein. The institutes' guidelines suggest that no more than 30 percent of your calories come from fat, that 55 to 60 percent come from carbohydrates and that no more than 15 percent come from protein. A gram of fat equals nine calories, while a gram of protein or carbohydrate equals four calories; therefore, if you eat 2,100 calories a day, you should consume approximately 60 grams of fat, 315 grams of carbohydrate and no more than 75 grams of protein daily. If you follow a lowfat/high-carbohydrate diet, your chance of developing heart disease, cancer and other life-threatening diseases may be considerably reduced.

The nutrition charts that accompany each of the lowfat/high-carbohydrate recipes in this book include the number of calories per serving, the number of grams of fat, carbohydrate and protein in a serving, and the percentage of calories derived from each of these nutrients. In addition, the charts provide the amount of calcium, iron and sodium per serving.

Calcium deficiency may be associated with periodontal disease — which attacks the mouth's bones and tissues, including the gums — in both men and women, and with osteoporosis, or bone shrinking and weakening, in the elderly. The deficiency may also contribute to high blood pressure. The recommended daily allowance for calcium is 800 milligrams a day for men and women. Pregnant and lactating women are advised to consume 1,200 milligrams daily; a National Institutes of Health consensus panel recommends that postmenopausal women consume 1,200 to 1,500 milligrams of calcium daily.

Although one way you can reduce your fat intake is to cut your consumption of red meat, you should make sure that you get your necessary iron from other sources. The Food and Nutrition Board of the National Academy of Sciences suggests a minimum of 10 milligrams of iron per day for men and 18 milligrams for women between the ages of 11 and 50.

High sodium intake is associated with high blood pressure. Most adults should restrict sodium intake to between 2,000 and 2,500 milligrams a day, according to the National Academy of Sciences. One way to keep sodium consumption in check is not to add table salt to food.

vitamin E may play a role in inhibiting the long-term cellular deterioration that occurs as part of the aging process and that may be due to oxidation. As a protector of cell membranes, vitamin E may also keep blood cells from breaking down. Among the good sources of vitamin E are oats, leafy green vegetables, whole-wheat products, nuts and virtually all vegetable oils except coconut oil.

Although your body does not make vitamin K directly, bacteria in your intestines can produce this vitamin, which reduces the amount you need from dietary sources. Used by your liver to make blood-clotting factors, vitamin K is found in spinach, kale, cabbage, cauliflower and liver, among other foods.

Measurable deficiencies of the fat-soluble vitamins are relatively uncommon, but no one who exercises regularly can afford to neglect foods that contain these vitamins. The recipes that follow are high in one or more of them.

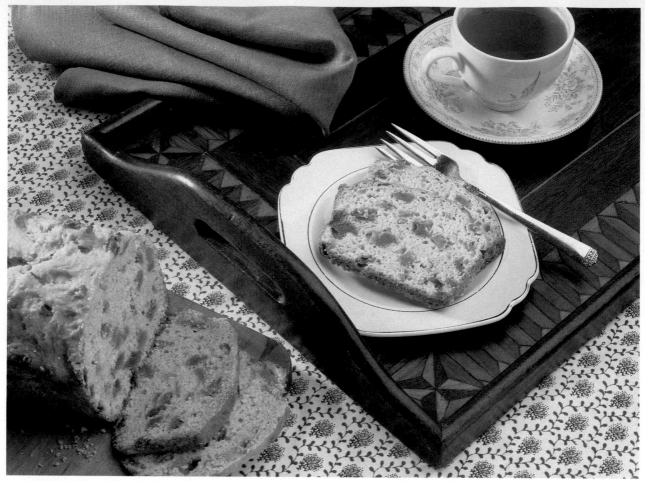

Winter Squash Bread

Breakfast

. . . .

WINTER SQUASH BREAD

This bread supplies nearly half your daily recommended vitamin A; a serving of a typical whole-wheat bread provides less than 2 percent.

CALORIES per slice	136
79% Carbohydrate	27 g
9% Protein	3 g
12% Fat	2 g
CALCIUM	40 mg
IRON	1 mg
SODIUM	146 mg

1 cup cooked Hubbard or other winter squash, or 1 small uncooked squash
6 ounces dried peaches
1/2 cup apple juice
Vegetable cooking spray
2 cups unbleached all-purpose flour, approximately

1/2 cup sugar
2 teaspoons baking powder
1 teaspoon ground allspice
1/2 teaspoon salt
1/4 teaspoon baking soda
2 eggs, beaten
1 tablespoon corn oil

If using uncooked squash, preheat the oven to 375° F. Using a large, heavy knife, carefully halve the squash. Place the halves cut side down on a foil-lined baking sheet and bake for 25 to 35 minutes, or until the flesh is tender when pierced with a knife. Reduce the oven temperature to 350° F, remove the squash from the oven and set aside to cool. Meanwhile, coarsely chop the peaches. Bring the apple juice to a boil in a small saucepan over medium heat. Remove the pan from the heat and stir in the peaches; set aside. When the squash is cool enough to handle, remove and discard the seeds and stringy membranes. Measure 1 cup of the cooked flesh into a small bowl and mash it with a fork; set aside. Reserve any remaining squash for another use.

Spray a 9 x 5-inch loaf pan with cooking spray and dust it lightly with flour. In a large bowl stir together 2 cups of flour, the sugar, baking powder, allspice, salt and baking soda, and make a well in the center. Add the peaches and apple juice, the eggs, oil and mashed squash, and mix just until blended. Turn the batter into the prepared pan and bake for 1 hour and 15 minutes, or until the loaf pulls away from the sides of the pan. Let the bread cool in the pan for 15 minutes, then turn it out onto a rack to cool completely. Cut the bread into sixteen 1/2-inch-thick slices.   Makes 16 servings

HOT FRUIT COMPOTE

A serving of this dish gives you about one fourth of your recommended daily vitamin C. The golden-yellow flesh of nectarines and plums comes from their beta carotene, a substance your body converts to vitamin A.

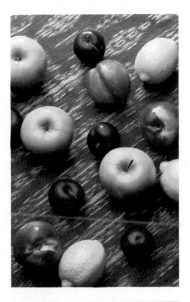

1 1/2 pounds black grapes, washed and stemmed (2 cups)	2 teaspoons vanilla extract
1 lemon, cut into wedges	2 Granny Smith apples
	2 nectarines
	2 plums

Purée the grapes in a food processor or blender. Strain the purée into a medium-size bowl, pressing with a rubber spatula to extract as much juice as possible; you should have about 1 cup of grape juice. Discard the pulp and seeds. Place the juice in a medium-size nonreactive saucepan, add the lemon wedges and vanilla and bring to a boil over medium heat. Meanwhile, core the apples and pit the nectarines and plums; do not peel the fruit. Cut the fruit into 1/2-inch-thick wedges and add it to the saucepan. Cover the pan, reduce the heat to low and simmer, stirring occasionally, for 10 to 15 minutes, or until the fruit is tender. Serve the compote hot, or cover and refrigerate it and serve it chilled. It will keep for 4 days in the refrigerator.   Makes 4 servings

CALORIES per serving	128
90% Carbohydrate	32 g
4% Protein	1 g
6% Fat	1 g
CALCIUM	16 mg
IRON	.4 mg
SODIUM	1 mg

CUCUMBER COOLER

All fluid milk and most dry milk in this country is fortified with vitamin D; a cup of buttermilk supplies about one fourth your daily allowance.

1 cup buttermilk	1 medium-size banana
One 2-inch cucumber section, peeled and cut into large chunks	4 mint sprigs
	1 ice cube

Combine all the ingredients in a food processor or blender and process until well blended. Pour the cooler into a tall glass and serve.   Makes 1 serving

CALORIES per serving	214
72%Carbohydrate	41 g
17% Protein	10 g
11% Fat	3 g
CALCIUM	307 mg
IRON	1 mg
SODIUM	260 mg

OLD-FASHIONED OATMEAL WAFFLES

CALORIES per serving	436
58% Carbohydrate	63 g
16% Protein	18 g
26% Fat	12 g
CALCIUM	336 mg
IRON	3 mg
SODIUM	517 mg

Since your body needs sunshine to synthesize vitamin D, you may need more dietary sources of this vitamin in winter, when you probably get less sunshine. The dairy products and eggs in these waffles supply good amounts of vitamin D, and you also get a healthy portion of oats, with their cholesterol-lowering fiber.

1 cup plain lowfat yogurt	2 teaspoons baking powder
1 cup unsweetened applesauce	2 eggs, separated
1 teaspoon vanilla extract	1/4 teaspoon salt
1 1/4 teaspoons ground cinnamon	1 cup skim milk
3/4 cup plus 2 tablespoons unbleached all-purpose flour	2 tablespoons butter, melted and cooled
2 cups rolled oats	Vegetable cooking spray (optional)

For the sauce, in a small bowl stir together the yogurt, applesauce, vanilla and 1 teaspoon of cinnamon; set aside. In a medium-size bowl stir together the flour, oats and baking powder; set aside. In a large bowl, using an electric mixer, beat the egg whites until frothy. Add the salt and continue to beat until the whites are stiff but not dry; set aside. Make a well in the center of the dry ingredients, add the milk, egg yolks and butter, and stir just until combined. Fold in the egg whites.

Preheat a nonstick waffle iron. (If your waffle iron does not have a nonstick surface, spray it with cooking spray before preheating it. Do not respray the hot iron.) Pour 1/3 cup of batter into the center of each section of the waffle iron and cook the waffles for about 4 minutes, or according to the manufacturer's instructions, until golden. Make 8 more individual waffles (filling the iron twice) in the same fashion. Divide the 12 individual waffles among 4 plates, top them with the yogurt sauce and dust them with the remaining cinnamon.

Makes 4 servings

TOMATO-LEMON BREAKFAST SHAKE

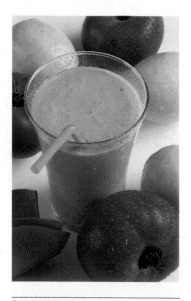

CALORIES per serving	263
66% Carbohydrate	45 g
21% Protein	14 g
13% Fat	4 g
CALCIUM	484 mg
IRON	2 mg
SODIUM	453 mg

Carotene is the provitamin, or precursor, of vitamin A that gives carrots their orange hue. The vitamin A content of carrots increases while they are in storage as long as they are kept in a cool, dark place.

1 large carrot	1 tablespoon sugar
1 cup plain lowfat yogurt	1 teaspoon grated lemon peel
2/3 cup drained canned tomatoes	

Trim and peel the carrot and cut it into 1/2-inch chunks. Place the carrot in a small saucepan with 1 cup of water and bring to a boil over high heat. Reduce the heat to low and simmer, partially covered, for 5 minutes. Drain the cooked carrot and place it in the refrigerator to cool for about 15 minutes.

Process the carrot in a food processor or blender until smoothly puréed. Add the yogurt, tomatoes, sugar and lemon peel, and process for 1 minute, or until smooth, scraping down the sides of the container with a rubber spatula if necessary. Pour the shake into a tall glass, over ice if desired, and serve.

Makes 1 serving

Lunch

ROSY RATATOUILLE

This version of a classic Provençal dish is rich in vitamins A and C.

1 pound sweet potatoes	4 garlic cloves, minced
3/4 pound baby beets	Two 14-ounce cans plum tomatoes
3/4 pound carrots	1/4 teaspoon dried basil
3/4 pound yellow squash	1/4 teaspoon dried thyme
1 tablespoon safflower oil	1 bay leaf
3 cups coarsely chopped onions	1/4 cup chopped fresh parsley

CALORIES per serving	261
73% Carbohydrate	46 g
11% Protein	7 g
16% Fat	5 g
CALCIUM	151 mg
IRON	4 mg
SODIUM	407 mg

Wash and trim the potatoes, beets, carrots and squash; peel all except the squash. Cut the potatoes, beets and squash into 1/4-inch-thick slices and halve the larger slices crosswise. Cut the carrots into 1-inch chunks.

Heat the oil in a Dutch oven or large heavy-gauge saucepan over medium heat. Add the onions and garlic and sauté, stirring constantly, for 10 minutes, or until the onions are translucent. Add the potatoes, the tomatoes with their liquid, the basil, thyme and bay leaf, and bring to a boil. Cover the pan, reduce the heat to low and simmer for 15 to 20 minutes, or until the potatoes are tender. Add the beets, carrots and parsley, and simmer for another 15 minutes. Add the squash, increase the heat to medium and cook, uncovered, for 5 minutes more, or until the squash is tender and the liquid is thickened. Remove and discard the bay leaf. Serve the ratatouille warm, or refrigerate it in a covered container for 3 to 4 hours and serve it cold.   Makes 4 servings

Note: If using mature beets, steam them whole for about 30 minutes, or until barely tender, then cool slightly, peel, slice and add them to the ratatouille.

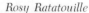

Rosy Ratatouille

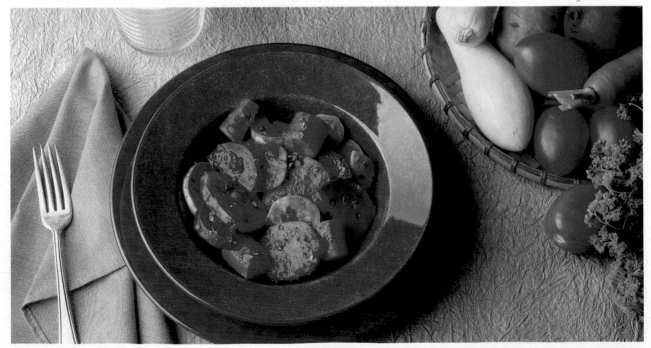

CREAMY CORN AND OAT SOUP

CALORIES per serving	154
73% Carbohydrate	30 g
15% Protein	6 g
12% Fat	2 g
CALCIUM	22 mg
IRON	1 mg
SODIUM	47 mg

Most grains lose up to 80 percent of their vitamin E when the bran and germ are removed in milling. When oats are milled, however, only the inedible hull is removed, so the oats remain a good source of vitamin E, thiamine and fiber.

2 cups fresh or frozen
  corn kernels
1 cup rolled oats
1/2 cup chopped onion
2 garlic cloves, minced

1/4 teaspoon pepper
Pinch of salt
2 tablespoons chopped
  fresh parsley

In a medium-size saucepan combine the corn, oats, onion, garlic, pepper, salt and 3 1/2 cups of water. Bring the mixture to a boil over medium heat, reduce the heat to low and simmer for 15 minutes. If a thinner soup is preferred, add up to 1/2 cup of water. Remove the pan from the heat, stir in 1 tablespoon of parsley and divide the soup among 4 bowls. Sprinkle the soup with the remaining parsley and serve.   Makes 4 servings

BUTTERNUT SQUASH SANDWICH

Almonds and peanuts, rich sources of vitamin E, should be eaten in moderation because of their high fat content. Here a sandwich spread made with peanut butter and almonds complements winter squash.

1 small butternut squash
4 whole blanched almonds
1/4 cup plain lowfat yogurt
2 teaspoons peanut butter
1 scallion, trimmed and chopped
Pinch of salt

Four 1/2-inch-thick slices dense
  whole-wheat bread
2 large Romaine lettuce leaves,
  torn into bite-size pieces
1 small tomato, sliced
1 ounce alfalfa sprouts

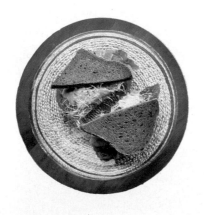

CALORIES per serving	262
58% Carbohydrate	41 g
17% Protein	12 g
25% Fat	8 g
CALCIUM	168 mg
IRON	3 mg
SODIUM	423 mg

Preheat the oven to 375° F. Line a baking sheet with aluminum foil. Using a large, heavy knife, carefully halve the squash. Place the squash halves cut side down on the baking sheet and bake for 25 minutes, or until the flesh is tender when pierced with a knife. Remove the squash from the oven and set aside to cool. Meanwhile, place the almonds in a small skillet and toast them over medium-high heat for 2 to 3 minutes, or until golden, tossing them frequently to prevent scorching. For the dressing, place the almonds in a food processor or blender (if using a blender, coarsely chop the almonds first) and process until puréed. Add the yogurt, peanut butter, scallion and salt, and process until blended; set aside.

    When the squash is cool enough to handle, remove and discard the seeds and stringy membranes. Peel one squash half and cut it lengthwise into four 1/4-inch-thick slices. (The remaining squash can be used in Winter Squash Bread, page 128.) Dip the squash slices in the dressing and set aside. Toast the bread and spread each piece with 1 tablespoon of dressing. Layer the lettuce, tomato, squash and sprouts on 2 pieces of toast and top with the remaining dressing. Place a second slice of toast on each sandwich, cut the sandwiches in half and serve immediately.   Makes 2 servings

BROCCOLI PIMIENTO SALAD

Dark green vegetables are rich sources of carotene: The broccoli in a serving of this salad supplies more than one fifth of your daily allowance of vitamin A. Broccoli is also a good source of calcium. The whole-wheat bread and corn oil contribute vitamin E to this dish.

1 pound broccoli
4 slices whole-wheat bread,
   cut into 1/2-inch cubes
3 whole canned pimientos
1/4 cup balsamic vinegar
2 teaspoons corn oil

2 teaspoons coarse-grain
   Dijon-style mustard
1 garlic clove, crushed and peeled
1/4 teaspoon dried tarragon
1/4 teaspoon pepper
Pinch of salt

CALORIES per serving	110
58% Carbohydrate	17 g
16% Protein	5 g
26% Fat	4 g
CALCIUM	61 mg
IRON	2 mg
SODIUM	206 mg

Preheat the oven to 375° F. Wash and trim the broccoli. Cut off the florets and cut the stems into 1-inch pieces; set aside. For the croutons, spread the bread cubes on a baking sheet and bake them for 5 to 10 minutes, or until golden. Meanwhile, bring 2 cups of water to a boil in a large saucepan over medium-high heat. Add the broccoli florets and stems and cook for 5 minutes, or until the stems are tender when pierced with a knife. Drain the broccoli, cool under cold water and set aside to drain thoroughly. Rinse and pat dry the pimientos and cut them into 1/4-inch-wide strips; set aside.

   For the dressing, in a small bowl whisk together the vinegar, oil, mustard, garlic, tarragon, pepper, salt and 2 tablespoons of water. Pat the broccoli dry, then place it in a large bowl with the pimiento. Add the croutons, pour on the dressing and toss to combine. Serve the salad immediately so that the croutons remain crisp.　　　　　Makes 4 servings

INDIAN SPICED PUMPKIN SOUP

Making pumpkin a once-a-year ingredient means you miss out on an excellent source of vitamin A. The high potassium, niacin, iron and calcium content of this vegetable are further incentives to use it more often. If you cook fresh pumpkin, toast and eat the seeds, an abundant source of vitamin E. A 2-pound pumpkin will yield the 2 cups of cooked pumpkin used here.

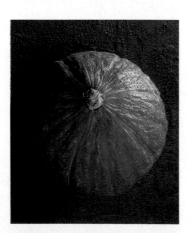

2 teaspoons butter
3/4 cup coarsely chopped onion
1 teaspoon ground coriander
1/2 teaspoon ground cumin
1/2 teaspoon ground turmeric
2 cups canned or cooked pumpkin

1/4 cup chopped fresh coriander
2 tablespoons brown sugar
2 tablespoons tomato paste
1 tablespoon peanut butter
1/4 teaspoon pepper
Pinch of salt

Melt the butter in a medium-size saucepan over medium heat. Add the onion and sauté for 3 to 4 minutes, or until light golden. Add the coriander, cumin and turmeric, and cook, stirring, for another minute. Add the pumpkin, coriander, sugar, tomato paste, peanut butter, pepper, salt and 3 cups of water, and stir gently to mix well. Bring the mixture to a boil, then cover the pan, reduce the heat to low and simmer the soup for about 30 minutes, or until the flavors are well blended. Ladle the soup into 4 bowls and serve. Makes 4 servings

CALORIES per serving	128
61% Carbohydrate	21 g
10% Protein	3 g
29% Fat	5 g
CALCIUM	55 mg
IRON	3 mg
SODIUM	146 mg

Dinner

· · · · · · · · · · · · ·

RICE-STUFFED ROASTED HENS WITH KALE

CALORIES per serving	361
50% Carbohydrate	44 g
28% Protein	25 g
22% Fat	9 g
CALCIUM	120 mg
IRON	3 mg
SODIUM	114 mg

Serving skinless poultry with generous portions of grains and vegetables maintains the proper carbohydrate-protein-fat balance. Brown rice, a whole grain, contributes vitamin E and several B vitamins.

1 tablespoon butter
1/2 cup chopped scallions
3 garlic cloves, chopped
1 1/2 cups cooked brown rice
1 cup cooked couscous
1 cup frozen corn kernels, thawed

1 tablespoon chopped fresh
  rosemary
2 small Cornish game hens (about
  3/4 pound each)
2 medium-size onions
1/2 pound kale

Preheat the oven to 425° F. Heat the butter in a small skillet over medium heat. Add the scallions and garlic and sauté for 3 minutes, then transfer to a medium-size bowl, add the rice, couscous, corn and rosemary and mix well.

Remove and discard any visible fat from the hens. Fill the hens with the rice mixture. Place any extra stuffing in a small baking dish and cover with foil. Line a roasting pan with foil. Peel the onions, cut them into 1/4-inch-thick slices and spread them in the pan. Place the hens in the pan and roast for 15 minutes, basting with pan juices. Meanwhile, wash and trim the kale. Add 3/4 cup of water to the roasting pan, reduce the heat to 350° F and place the dish of stuffing in the oven. Cook the stuffing and the hens for 30 minutes, or until the juices run clear when the thigh joints are pierced with a knife.

Remove the dish of stuffing from the oven. Transfer the hens to a serving

Rice-Stuffed Roasted Hens with Kale

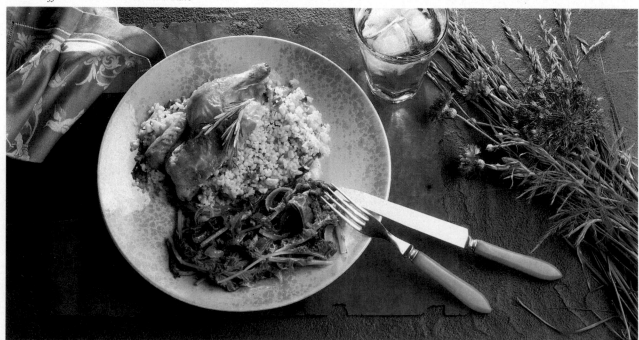

platter and cover loosely with foil. Scrape the onions and pan juices into a medium-size saucepan and bring to a boil over medium-high heat. Add the kale and cover the pan. Reduce the heat to medium low and simmer the kale, stirring occasionally, for 10 minutes, or until tender. Divide the stuffing and kale among 4 plates. Split the Cornish hens, place one half on each plate and serve. Remove the skin from the hens before eating.   Makes 4 servings

SUMMER CANTALOUPE SOUP

Puréed sweet potato, not cream, thickens this vitamin A-rich soup.

2 medium-size cantaloupes
1 pound sweet potatoes, trimmed
1 cup skim milk
1 cup plain lowfat yogurt

1/4 cup frozen apple
  juice concentrate
1 tablespoon grated lemon peel
8 mint sprigs

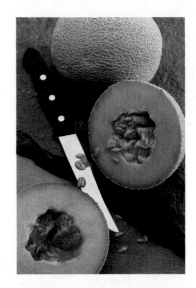

Halve and seed the cantaloupes. Spoon the flesh into a food processor or blender, process until liquefied and transfer to a large bowl; set aside. Place the potatoes in a medium-size saucepan with cold water to cover and bring to a boil over medium-high heat. Reduce the heat to low, partially cover the pan and simmer for 45 minutes, or until tender; drain and set aside to cool.

When the potatoes are cool enough to handle, peel them, cut them into large chunks and process until puréed. Gradually add the cantaloupe juice, the milk, yogurt, apple juice concentrate and lemon peel, and process until well blended. Return the soup to the bowl and add 4 mint sprigs, crushing them gently with a wooden spoon to release their flavor. Cover the bowl and refrigerate the soup overnight. To serve, remove the mint, ladle the soup into 4 bowls and garnish each serving with a fresh mint sprig.   Makes 4 servings

CALORIES per serving	269
81% Carbohydrate	57 g
13% Protein	9 g
6% Fat	2 g
CALCIUM	233 mg
IRON	1 mg
SODIUM	111 mg

CAVIAR-OLIVE PASTA SALAD

Skim milk, because it is fortified, and caviar, because it comes from fish, are both excellent sources of vitamin D.

6 ounces fusilli or rotelle
  (spiral) pasta
1/2 cup lowfat, low-sodium
  cottage cheese (1%)
1/4 cup packed fresh
  parsley sprigs

2 tablespoons coarsely
  chopped scallion
1/4 cup skim milk
Pinch of pepper
8 large pitted black olives,
  slivered
1 teaspoon red caviar

Bring a large pot of water to a boil, add the pasta and cook for 10 minutes, or according to the package directions until al dente. Drain the pasta, cool under cold water and set aside to drain thoroughly. For the sauce, process the cottage cheese, parsley and scallion in a food processor or blender for 1 to 2 minutes, or until smooth, scraping down the sides of the container with a rubber spatula as necessary. Add the milk and pepper and process for another 5 seconds. Transfer the pasta and sauce to a large bowl and toss to coat the pasta with sauce. Scatter the olives and caviar on top and toss the salad again just before serving.   Makes 4 servings

CALORIES per serving	198
69% Carbohydrate	34 g
19% Protein	9 g
12% Fat	3 g
CALCIUM	57 mg
IRON	2 mg
SODIUM	107 mg

WILD RICE SALAD WITH WALNUT-ORANGE DRESSING

CALORIES per serving	243
59% Carbohydrate	38 g
14% Protein	9 g
27% Fat	8 g
CALCIUM	35 mg
IRON	3 mg
SODIUM	45 mg

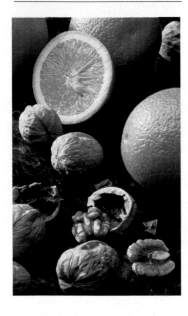

Cooking oils are the richest dietary sources of vitamin E. Brussels sprouts contain some vitamins A and E and are rich in vitamin K.

1 cup wild rice	1/2 teaspoon orange extract
One 10-ounce package frozen Brussels sprouts, thawed	1/4 teaspoon pepper
	Pinch of salt
1/3 cup freshly squeezed orange juice	1 cup slivered red bell pepper
	2 tablespoons chopped fresh mint
2 tablespoons walnut oil	4 large Romaine lettuce leaves

Bring 3 1/2 cups of water to a boil in a medium-size saucepan over medium-high heat. Add the rice, reduce the heat to low and simmer, partially covered, for 45 minutes. Halve the sprouts and set aside to drain on paper towels.

Remove the pan of rice from the heat and stir in the orange juice, oil, orange extract, pepper and salt. Stir in the Brussels sprouts, bell pepper and mint. Let the mixture cool slightly, then transfer it to a large bowl, cover with plastic wrap and refrigerate it overnight, stirring occasionally. To serve, line a platter with Romaine and mound the salad on top.   Makes 4 servings

GREEN TAMALE PIE

Color is an indicator of vitamin A in cornmeal just as it is in corn and other fresh vegetables: White cornmeal has no significant vitamin A, while yellow meal has a considerable quantity.

2 cups frozen lima beans, thawed	1/2 cup corn kernels
1 cup washed, trimmed spinach	1 cup coarsely chopped green bell pepper
2 scallions, trimmed and coarsely chopped	Vegetable cooking spray
2 tablespoons tomato paste	1 1/2 cups yellow cornmeal
1 garlic clove	Pinch of salt
4 teaspoons chili powder	1/4 cup grated Cheddar cheese

CALORIES per serving	230
75% Carbohydrate	43 g
14% Protein	8 g
11% Fat	3 g
CALCIUM	64 mg
IRON	3 mg
SODIUM	148 mg

Place the beans, spinach, scallions, tomato paste, garlic and 2 teaspoons of chili powder in a food processor or blender and process for 1 to 2 minutes, or until puréed, scraping down the sides of the container with a rubber spatula as necessary. Stir in the corn and bell pepper and set aside.

Preheat the oven to 350° F. Spray a heavy-gauge ovenproof skillet (preferably cast iron) with cooking spray; set aside. In a medium-size saucepan over medium heat, combine the cornmeal, salt, remaining chili powder and 2 1/2 cups of cold water and, cook, stirring constantly, for 2 to 3 minutes, or until the mixture thickens and comes to a boil. Remove the pan from the heat and spread two thirds of the cornmeal mixture in the prepared skillet. Spoon the lima bean purée over it, top with the remaining cornmeal mixture and sprinkle the pie with cheese. Bake the tamale pie for 30 minutes, or until the cheese is melted and the top is lightly browned. To serve, cut the pie into 6 wedges.
                                                            Makes 6 servings

Desserts

APRICOT AND PRUNE FLANS

Using eggs and milk together gives you both calcium and vitamin D, which work in tandem to keep your bones strong and healthy. Apricots and prunes, excellent sources of vitamin A, also provide potassium, an important mineral to replenish when you are exercising strenuously.

3/4 cup dried apricot halves

3/4 cup pitted prunes

2 eggs

1/3 cup honey

2/3 cup unbleached
  all-purpose flour

1 3/4 cups skim milk

CALORIES per serving	246
81% Carbohydrate	52 g
11% Protein	7 g
8% Fat	2 g
CALCIUM	118 mg
IRON	2 mg
SODIUM	64 mg

Place the apricots and prunes in a medium-size bowl, add boiling water to cover and set aside to soak for 1 hour.

Preheat the oven to 350° F. For the custard, in a small bowl beat together the eggs and honey until smooth. Gradually whisk in the flour, then stir in the milk. Drain the fruit and divide it among six 8-ounce custard cups or ramekins. Divide the custard among the cups and bake for 1 hour, or until the custard is set and golden brown around the edges. Serve the flans warm, or cover them, refrigerate until well chilled and serve cold.   Makes 6 servings

Apricot and Prune Flans

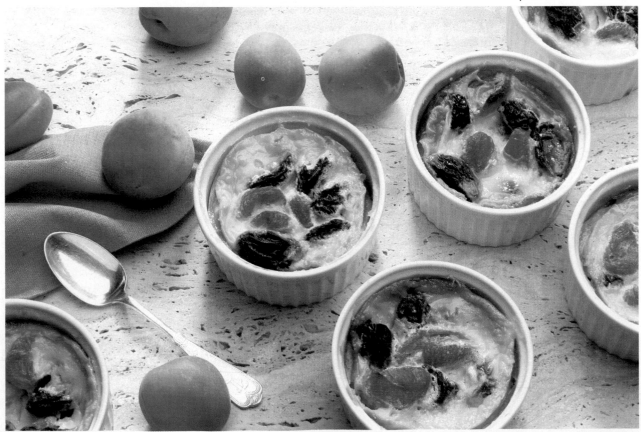

CALORIES per serving	102
69% Carbohydrate	19 g
6% Protein	2 g
25% Fat	3 g
CALCIUM	25 mg
IRON	1 mg
SODIUM	7 mg

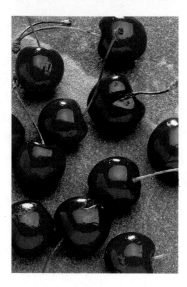

CALORIES per serving	259
77% Carbohydrate	51 g
11% Protein	7 g
12% Fat	3 g
Calcium	120 mg
IRON	1 mg
SODIUM	91 mg

CALORIES per serving	199
81% Carbohydrate	42 g
18% Protein	10 g
1% Fat	.2 g
CALCIUM	224 mg
IRON	1 mg
SODIUM	116 mg

CHERRY-ALMOND SOUP

Sixty percent of your dietary vitamin E comes from oils and fat, and about 10 percent from fruits and vegetables.

8 almond-flavored tea bags
2 teaspoons vanilla extract
1 tablespoon honey

2 cups pitted fresh sweet cherries,
  or frozen unsweetened cherries
1/4 cup nonbutterfat sour dressing

Bring 1 quart of water to a boil. Place the tea bags in a heatproof bowl, pour the boiling water over them, cover and let steep for 15 minutes. Remove and discard the tea bags and stir in the vanilla and honey; set aside. Place the cherries in a food processor or blender and process until puréed, then stir the cherry purée into the tea. Cover the bowl and refrigerate the soup for at least 4 hours, or until thoroughly chilled. To serve, divide the soup among 4 bowls and top each serving with 1 tablespoon of sour dressing.   Makes 4 servings

CARROT RICE PUDDING

This old-fashioned dish fulfills your daily requirement for vitamin A while providing good amounts of vitamins D and E.

1 cup carrot juice
1 cup skim milk
1/4 cup sugar
3 tablespoons instant tapioca

2 eggs, beaten
1 cup cooked brown rice
1/2 cup grated carrot
1/3 cup dark raisins

Bring enough water to a simmer in the bottom of a double boiler so that the water will not touch the top pan. For the custard, in the top pan stir together the carrot juice, milk, sugar, tapioca and eggs until well blended, then cook, without stirring, over the simmering water for 5 minutes. Increase the heat to medium-high to bring the water in the bottom pan to a boil, and cook the custard, whisking constantly, for another 5 minutes. Remove the top pan from the heat and stir the rice, carrot and raisins into the custard. Turn the mixture into a serving dish and let cool at room temperature for about 1 hour, or cover and refrigerate for 2 to 3 hours and serve cold.   Makes 4 servings

MANDARIN ORANGE WHIP

Evaporated skimmed milk, fortified with vitamins A and D, is rich-tasting but contains less than 1 gram of fat per cup.

4 cups drained canned mandarin
  orange sections
3 tablespoons brown sugar
1 package unflavored gelatin
1 cup evaporated skimmed milk

2 teaspoons lime juice
1 teaspoon grated lime peel
1 teaspoon vanilla extract
2 egg whites

Place 2 cups of oranges in a food processor or blender and process until liquefied, then transfer to a small saucepan and heat over medium-low heat for 5 minutes, or just until tepid. Add the sugar and gelatin, and stir until the gelatin dissolves. Remove the pan from the heat. Add the remaining oranges, the milk, lime juice, lime peel and vanilla extract, and stir to combine.

In a large bowl, using an electric mixer, beat the egg whites until stiff but not dry. Fold the whites into the orange mixture, breaking up any large clumps of egg white, and stir just until mixed. Transfer the mixture to a 1 1/2-quart soufflé dish or divide it among 4 individual dessert dishes. Cover and refrigerate for 3 to 4 hours, or until set. Makes 4 servings

MOROCCAN-STYLE FRUITED COUSCOUS

Couscous, a granular semolina product, is usually cooked with meat and vegetables but, like rice, also makes a good dessert. Yogurt adds calcium, and the almonds are a good source of vitamin E.

CALORIES per serving	215
70% Carbohydrate	37 g
19% Protein	6 g
11% Fat	4 g
CALCIUM	89 mg
IRON	1 mg
SODIUM	26 mg

1/3 cup golden raisins
12 whole toasted almonds
5 dried apricot halves, slivered
1 cup apple juice

1/3 cup instant couscous
1/2 cup plain lowfat yogurt
1 tablespoon brown sugar
1/2 teaspoon almond extract

In a small bowl toss together the raisins, almonds and apricots. Bring the apple juice to a boil in a medium-size saucepan over medium heat. Stir in the couscous and cook, stirring, for 2 minutes, or until thickened. Remove the pan from the heat and stir in the yogurt, sugar and almond extract. Divide the couscous among 4 bowls and top it with the fruit mixture. Makes 4 servings

CARROT-APPLESAUCE CAKE SQUARES

Egg yolks, unlike produce, do not reveal their vitamin A content by the intensity of their color: A pale yolk has as much vitamin A as a dark yellow one. The yolk also contains all the egg's vitamin D.

Vegetable cooking spray
1 1/4 cups unbleached all-purpose
  flour, approximately
1/4 cup packed brown sugar
2 teaspoons baking powder
1/2 teaspoon ground cinnamon

2 eggs
1/2 cup unsweetened applesauce
3 tablespoons walnut oil
1 cup cooked brown rice
  (1/3 cup raw)
1 cup grated carrots

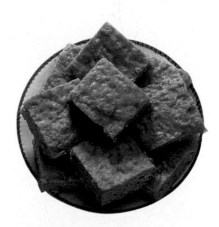

Preheat the oven to 400° F. Spray an 8 x 8-inch baking pan with cooking spray and lightly flour it; set aside. In a medium-size bowl stir together 1 1/4 cups of flour, the sugar, baking powder and cinnamon, and make a well in the center. In a small bowl beat together the eggs, applesauce and oil. Pour this mixture into the dry ingredients, add the rice and carrots and stir until the dry ingredients are moistened. Spread the batter in the pan and bake for 40 minutes, or until the top is lightly browned and a toothpick inserted into the cake comes out dry. (The cake will rise very little.) Let the cake cool in the pan on a rack for 15 minutes, then cut it into 9 squares. Makes 9 servings

CALORIES per square	183
61% Carbohydrate	28 g
8% Protein	4 g
31% Fat	6 g
CALCIUM	69 mg
IRON	1 mg
SODIUM	117 mg

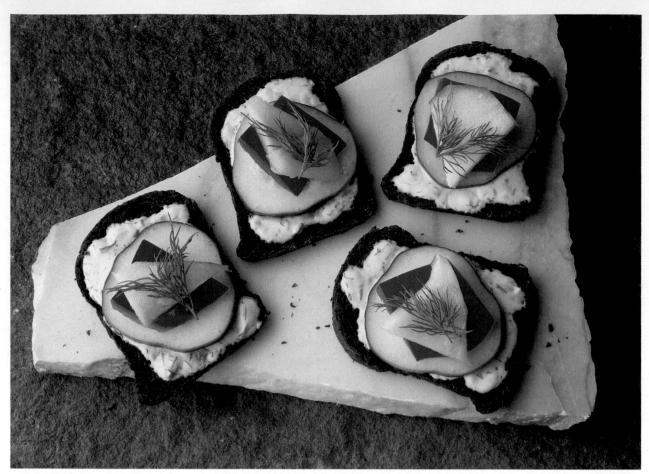

Scandinavian-style Canapés

Snacks

. . . .

SCANDINAVIAN-STYLE CANAPES

Fish are the only animals that can manufacture vitamin D in the absence of ultraviolet light: Fatty fish such as sablefish, salmon and herring are the richest sources of this vitamin.

CALORIES per serving	123
61% Carbohydrate	20 g
18% Protein	6 g
21% Fat	3 g
CALCIUM	73 mg
IRON	1 mg
SODIUM	325 mg

1/4 cup plain lowfat yogurt
2 teaspoons Dijon-style mustard
1 tablespoon chopped fresh dill, plus 16 dill sprigs
16 slices cocktail pumpernickel bread
Sixteen 1/4-inch-thick cucumber slices
1 red bell pepper, cut into sixteen 1-inch squares
2 ounces smoked sablefish, cut into 16 pieces

In a small bowl stir together the yogurt, mustard and chopped dill. Spread the bread with the yogurt mixture. Place a cucumber slice and a bell pepper square on each piece of bread and top with a piece of fish and a dill sprig. Arrange the canapés on a platter and serve. If not serving immediately, cover the platter with plastic wrap and refrigerate.   Makes 4 servings

CHOPPED LIVER SPREAD

Chicken liver is a good source of all the fat-soluble vitamins, especially vitamin A, which is stored in the liver. When chopped liver is prepared without added butter or chicken fat, it is a relatively lowfat appetizer.

CALORIES per serving	152
6% Carbohydrate	22 g
15% Protein	6 g
29% Fat	5 g
CALCIUM	10 mg
IRON	3 mg
SODIUM	143 mg

6 ounces chicken livers, washed
  and trimmed
2 tablespoons chopped shallots
2 tablespoons plain lowfat yogurt

2 teaspoons Dijon-style mustard
1/4 teaspoon pepper
Pinch of salt
48 small low-sodium crackers

Bring 1 1/2 cups of water to a boil in a small saucepan over medium-high heat. Add the chicken livers, reduce the heat to medium-low, cover and simmer for 5 minutes, stirring occasionally to ensure even cooking. Drain the livers and set aside to cool, then quarter them, place them in a food processor or blender and process for about 30 seconds, or until smooth. Add the shallots, yogurt, mustard, pepper and salt and process for another 30 seconds. Spread 1 teaspoon of chopped liver on each cracker.   Makes 8 servings

STUFFED TOMATOES

The large, yellow-fleshed rutabaga contains twice as much vitamin C, calcium and potassium as its relative the turnip.

1 large rutabaga (about 18
  ounces)
1 1/4 cups chopped onions
1 tablespoon chopped fresh
  parsley
1 tablespoon plus 1 teaspoon
  vegetable oil

2 tablespoons tomato paste
1/4 teaspoon pepper, or to taste
Pinch of salt
8 fresh plum tomatoes (about
    1 3/4 pounds total weight)

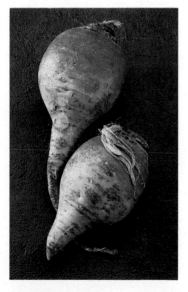

Using a sharp knife, pare a 1/4-inch thickness of skin from the rutabaga. (Rutabagas are heavily waxed for the market, so you must pare enough to remove the wax as well as the outer skin.) Cut the rutabaga into small chunks and grate it in a food processor using the grating blade, or quarter the rutabaga and grate it by hand; you should have about 5 cups. Steam the grated rutabaga in a vegetable steamer over boiling water for 15 to 20 minutes, or just until the raw taste is gone; the rutabaga should still be crisp. Transfer the cooked rutabaga to a large bowl and set aside to cool.

  Mix the cooled rutabaga with the onions and parsley. Heat 2 teaspoons of oil in a medium-size skillet over medium-high heat, add the rutabaga mixture and cook, stirring occasionally, for 2 to 3 minutes, or until the vegetables begin to brown. Add the remaining oil and cook, stirring, for another 2 to 3 minutes. Stir in the tomato paste, pepper and salt, remove the pan from the heat and set aside to cool. Meanwhile, cut off and discard 1/4 inch from the stem end of each tomato. Carefully scoop out the flesh, leaving a 1/4-inch-thick shell, and mix the tomato flesh with the rutabaga mixture. Stuff the tomatoes with the filling, mounding it at the top, and serve. Or wrap the tomatoes, refrigerate them until well chilled and cut them in half lengthwise to reveal the filling.

      Makes 4 servings

CALORIES per serving	139
58% Carbohydrate	22 g
10% Protein	4 g
32% Fat	5 g
CALCIUM	80 mg
IRON	2 mg
SODIUM	136 mg

PROP CREDITS

Cover: Leotard–Marika, San Diego, Calif., tights–Dance France LTD., Santa Monica, Calif.; page 6: jacket–Naturalife, New York City; sweat shirt–The Gap, San Francisco, Calif.; page 24: tank top–Athletic Style, New York City; page 29: sneakers–Avia, Alexandria, Va., Reebok International LTD., Avon, Mass., The Rockport Company, Marlboro, Mass.; pages 36-61: leotard, capri pants, trunks–Marika, courtesy of The Weekend Exercise Co., San Diego, Calif., sneakers–Nautilus Athletic Footwear, Inc., Greenville, S.C., wrist weights–Triangle Health and Fitness Systems, Morrisville, N.C.; pages 64-69: shirt–Athletic Style, New York City, shorts–Naturalife, New York City, sneakers–Reebok International, LTD., Avon, Mass.; pages 74-97: all swimsuits and equipment–The Finals, Port Jervis, N.Y.; page 98: leotard, tights, trunks–Marika, courtesy of The Weekend Exercise Co., San Diego, Calif.; pages 102-123: leotard, tights–Dance France, LTD., Santa Monica, Calif., mat–AMF American, Jefferson, Iowa, shirt–Calvin Klein Menswear, New York City, sweat pants–The Gap, San Francisco, Calif.; page 128: tablecloth–Pierre Deux, New York City; page 131: bowl, plate, glass–Ad Hoc Softwares, New York City.

ACKNOWLEDGMENTS

Our thanks to E.C. Frederick, president of Exeter Research, Inc., Brentwood, N.H., for his research assistance

The One-Mile Walk Test on page 21 was reprinted courtesy of The Rockport Company, ©1987 The Rockport Company

All cosmetics and grooming products supplied by Clinique Labs, Inc., New York City

Nutrition analysis provided by Hill Nutrition Associates, Fayetteville, N.Y.

Off-camera warm-up equipment: rowing machine supplied by Precor USA, Redmond, Wash.; Tunturi stationary bicycle supplied by Amerec Corp., Bellevue, Wash.

Washing machine and dryer supplied by White-Westinghouse, Columbus, Ohio

Index prepared by Ian Tucker

Production by Giga Communications

PHOTOGRAPHY CREDITS

Exercise photographs by Andrew Eccles; water workouts photographs by John Zimmerman; food photographs by Steven Mays, Rebus, Inc.

ILLUSTRATION CREDITS

Page 9, illustration: David Flaherty; page 10, illustration: Brian Sisco, Tammi Colichio; page 15, illustration: David Flaherty, chart: Brian Sisco; page 16, illustration: Brian Sisco, Tammi Colichio; page 21, chart: Brian Sisco, Tammi Colichio; page 23, illustration: Tammi Colichio; pages 62-63, charts: Brian Sisco, Tammi Colichio.

INDEX